HEAVEN LIES WITH

OR

YOGA GAVE ME
SUPERIOR HEALTH

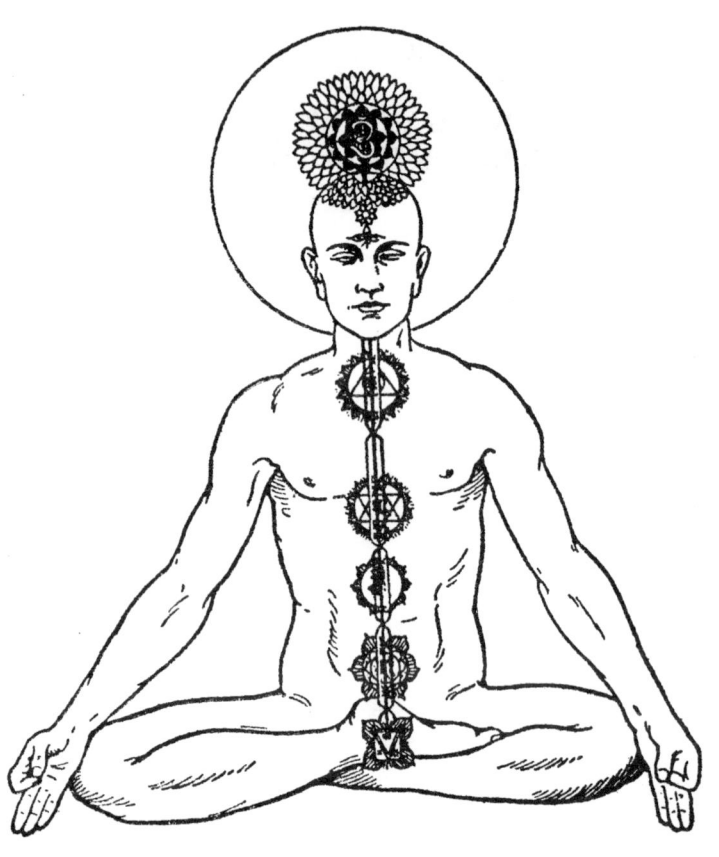

THE LOCATION OF THE CHAKRAS

HEAVEN LIES WITHIN US

By
THEOS BERNARD
Author of
" *Land of a Thousand Buddhas* "

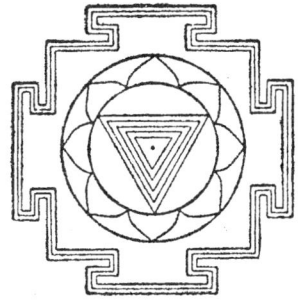

Second Impression

Essence of Health
Box 1129
Wandsbeck
3631
South Africa
essence@iafrica.com
http://www.Essenceofhealth.net

First Published in USA. **1939**
Published in **Britain 1941**
Reprinted in South Africa 1975

This Edition 2002
Copyright Essence of Health

ISBN 0-9584461-1-3

Essence of Health
Box 1129
Wandsbeck
3631
South Africa
essence@iaffica.com
http://www.Essenceofhealth.net

To
MY FATHER

The publishers regret to announce the death of the author in the following circumstances, as related by G. A. Bernard, the author's father.

"In 1947, Theos Bernard was on a mission to the KI monastery in western Tibet in search of some special manuscripts. While on his way, rioting broke out among the Hindus and Moslems in that section of the hills; all Moslems including children and women in the little village from which Theos departed were killed.

"The Hindus then proceeded into the mountains in pursuit of the Moslems who had accompanied Theos as guides and muleteers. These Moslems, it is reported, learning of the killings, escaped, leaving Theos and his Tibetan boy alone on the trail. It is further reported that both were shot and their bodies thrown in the river.

"To date we have not been able to get authentic information on the entire circumstances of his death, nor have we any line on the effects Theos had with him. That region of Tibet is so remote that it is unlikely that we shall ever learn the full deatails.

CONTENTS

CHAPTER		PAGE
I.	How My Interest in Yoga Began	13
II.	Some Preliminaries	27
III.	I Make a Start	37
IV.	I Go to India, the Home of Yoga	48
V.	The Meaning of Yoga	57
VI.	Some Rules for the Yogic Disciple	70
VII.	"More in Heaven and Earth..."	77
VIII.	Apprenticeship of the Mind	89
IX.	Consciousness	99
X.	Sights and Experiences in India	115
XI.	More about the Science of Breath	133
XII.	Importance of Pranayama	144
XIII.	Exercises to Cure Diseases and to Extend Youth	154
XIV.	Contrasts in India	170
XV.	Important Postures in Yoga	180
XVI.	Standing on One's Head, etc.	191
XVII.	About Mudras	199
XVIII.	Mystic and Eternal Aspects of Yoga	215
XIX.	Kundalini	230
XX.	My Final Initiation	243
	Index	253

The drawings at the heads of the chapters have all been reproduced from an original handwritten Tibetan manuscript on the practice of Yoga which was given to the author by his teacher.

FOREWORD

IN the preparation of this book, it has been my desire to leave a record of an American, one of my own creed and culture, who has tasted and lived the Way of Life taught by Yoga and can personally attest to every one of its claims.

It has been nearly two years since my return from the Orient, and from the very moment I set foot on the shores of America I have had to live at a "mile-a-minute" pace. This has been on account of a series of material circumstances in which we in this Western World unsuspectingly and frequently become involved. Yet I have conducted my every hour of action and have maintained a frame of mind and an attitude toward life according to this new way which has now become a part of my very being.

Experience has proven to me that this Way of Life will beyond any doubt enable one to touch greater depths of consciousness and get much more out of life through one's everyday experiences. These experiences will no longer be lost, but will be converted into blessings. If one is unsuccessful in attempting to follow the Path herein set forth, it will not be because Yoga does not show the right direction; it will be due rather to my own inadequacy in conveying its hidden principles. For Yoga is a "living philosophy," and virtually beyond the scope of the printed word.

It should be understood that in India everything is wrapped in the veils of religion. Nothing is done without some religious rite or ritual. At times one will find the most rational minds there revealing blind faith. This holds true from the highest to the lowest. I recall a visit to a very wealthy Indian business man who was as "up and coming" as a New York stock broker, but even he would get up at four in the morning to take his bath in the Sacred Ganges. When you consider the fact that even the lay people fill their lives with ritual, it is easy to understand how much formality there is among the devout.

This made it necessary that I go to India as a disciple and not as a research scholar to compare and weigh their teachings in the light of Western science. It was my purpose to try to get behind the forms of worship in order to discover for myself the true value that was to be found in the various practices of Yoga. Before I left America, I had a fair knowledge concerning the teachings and practices which I had been able to glean from personal sources and from poring over a tremendous mass of confused literature written by scholars without personal experience.

As will be seen from my study, I had made considerable progress with the practices themselves. I had gone far enough to know that the methods in and of themselves would not bring the student to the mental and spiritual realization for which he could rightfully hope. It was necessary to follow some regulated sequence, and this could only be done under the guidance of a teacher. This meant a journey to India, the home of Yoga. There was no place in America where one could go for such training nor was there any one whose knowledge was sufficient to guide one. When I was graduated from Law School, I entered Columbia University to study for a doctor's degree in the field of philosophy as a background for my future work, because it seemed to me as an Occidental that I should first familiarize myself with our own philosophical heritage.

When I began my studies in India, the first dictum of my teacher was to forget everything that I had learned. The purpose of this was to remove all prejudices and enable me to keep an open mind and heart. In order to do this I had to go through endless ritualistic forms which were obviously as useless to me as they would appear to any reader. Only thus could I become one of them, a devotee and a disciple, which was my earnest desire. At times I must confess it was exceedingly difficult to maintain a rational mind, as the rituals themselves were intended to erase the mind. Yet I had to pass through these experiences, in some instances to learn no more than I already knew and then offer thanks to the one who had conducted the Puja (worship). In any case, this was all essential in order to penetrate the veils of Maya.

In the writing of my experiences, I have tried not to burden the reader with an over-emphasis on this ritualistic side, which would require a book in itself. The purpose of this volume is primarily to reveal the various practices of Yoga in some organized fashion, so that an independent student may have a basis on which he can proceed alone, and I have woven the material around my own personal story. This, I hope, will instil confidence and make it easier for those who desire, to adapt this Way of Life to their own needs.

I have related the difficulties and rigid discipline that I had to follow. In order to cast a little light on the purpose of these practices, I have given some of the philosophical theory. It would be unintelligible as well as wearisome if I adhered to the chronological order in which this material has been gathered, as I have picked it up here and there from endless sources during the course of my travels and study in India and Tibet.

One thought in particular that my teachers gave me should be passed on to others in order to help them in their future readings and studies. At the very beginning I was told there were " no mysteries in Yoga " ; that everything could be explained ; that all the technique was based upon some logical foundation as well as supported by a rational philosophical scheme of life ; that everything was according to Law ; that nothing was without reason.

All that was required of me was an open mind. In due course, it was promised, I would come to understand the meaning behind the externals. It was not for me to find a reason for things in the beginning. My knowledge was not yet full enough for that. From my own experience, I can assure the prospective student of Yoga that the " open-minded policy " is the first essential and if he will follow it, he will likewise find there are no idle gestures.

Many will perhaps feel that they are too old to begin the practice of Yoga. This is quite wrong. It is taught in India that it is never too late to begin and that the slightest effort spent is never lost. There is authentic record in India of a famed Yogi who did not begin the practice until he was past fifty, and lived to be over two hundred years of age. A Yogi is not so much interested in finding the Fountain of Youth as he is in continuing the Spirit of Youth to the very end. There is nothing that will fill the human heart with more cheer than the practice of Yoga. It will give one the greatest joy, and help him to face life in its most dire aspects with understanding and courage. The Spirit of Youth will be a lifetime possession.

To the many authors who have aided me by their contributions to the subject I offer my thanks. To my teachers with whom I have sat and talked for hours about the Art of Yoga I am for all time deeply indebted for their eager assistance, their infinite patience, and their generous stimulation and encouragement.

THEOS BERNARD.

BEVERLY HILLS, CALIFORNIA.
August 1, 1939.

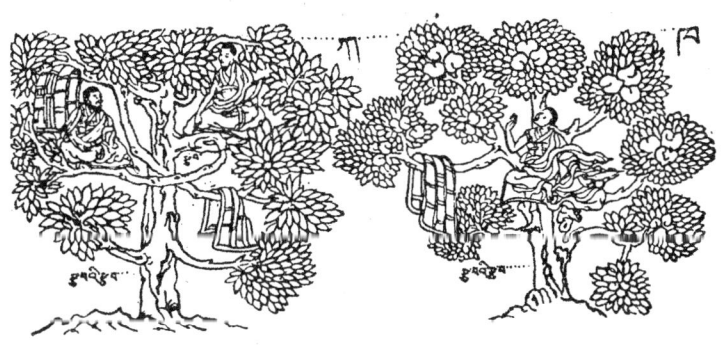

CHAPTER I

HOW MY INTEREST IN YOGA BEGAN

I

I OVERHEARD the doctor speaking to my nurse. He said : " He will not live."
I had been in the University Infirmary for several weeks with a severe attack of inflammatory rheumatism. And now my heart was beginning to fail me. I was singularly sensitive to the atmosphere, which was becoming increasingly tense. The general impression it conveyed to me was that it was only a matter of time. In the meanwhile, they would keep me sufficiently doped with morphine, so that the agony itself would not rob me of my last breath.

By now the condition had become so acute that every joint of my body was swollen. Indeed, all of my body had become so sensitive to pain that not even the sheets were allowed to touch me. A wall of pillows was built all around me, and the sheets were stretched tight above me. The attendants could not enter the room without causing me pain ; I was conscious of every step they took across the floor. Above all, I dreaded even the thought of a shot in my arm of mercurochrome, which it was presumed might help me. It was rather new on the market at the time, and, I suppose, I was just as good a guinea pig as could be found ; so why not experiment? Was I not as good as dead? The reaction to these shots was almost beyond my power of endurance. After a few minutes I would feel cold chills coming on. They would pack hot water bottles alongside of me and then pile on woollen blankets. Soon the chills would break, and the body would begin to shake like a chicken with its head cut off. The bed would vibrate, while they would try to hold me still in my last earthly shiver, but to no avail. There was nothing for me to do but to learn to take it, as the expression goes.

Bad as it was, the physical pain did not compare with the horrors that filled my imagination. For until this illness I seemed to be a perfect physical specimen, and now to contemplate the prospect of being an invalid for the rest of my days, even if I should miraculously survive, was too much for me. As the weeks rolled by and spring arrived, I could watch my fellow classmates through the hospital window training on the athletic field for the spring meet. From my earliest childhood I had always held to a strict discipline, with the dream of becoming some day a fine athlete. I had earned every available letter in High School; it was my ambition to continue in my favourite sports of running and swimming, as well as in my hobby of mountain climbing.

All in all, there was nothing here to cheer my imagination, and my mother, a discerning woman, made up her mind to take me back to my home town, which was ominously called Tombstone.

The doctors fulminated, forbade her to remove me, threatening the most dire consequences if she persisted in her course. But my mother was no slave to regulations, and when I pleaded with her to take me away, on the ground that I could endure no longer the cold mechanical care of the hospital and that I didn't care what happened to me, she promptly sized up the situation and, in the face of the doctors' protests, took matters into her own hands. She had a friend drive up to the hospital and I was removed, but not before she signed releases to free the doctors and the University from all blame. These releases were my freedom, and under my

How My Interest in Yoga Began

mother's hourly attention week after week, I began to recover. As long as I live, I want to say in passing, I shall never forget the seventy-eight-mile ride home over that dusty corrugated Arizona highway. I rarely pass over our paved boulevards of to-day without appreciation.

For months I was unable to consume any food except what I could suck through a glass tube, as it was impossible for me to turn my body and raise my head sufficiently to eat. Those early days of convalescence were like trying to learn how to live again. In the beginning I had to be carried to my chair, and was only strong enough to sit up about half an hour. It was an event when I was able to take three or four steps necessary to walk to the chair. My mother must have experienced some of the past joys in watching her child grow up, as I learned anew the early processes of life.

Even after I was able to be up all day, it was still several months before I had sufficient strength to take full care of myself. My deepest grief at the time was having to give up school for a whole year, and there was nothing to reconcile me to this loss. My mother had been in ill health virtually all my life, and through the years she had read many books which dealt for the most part with Eastern philosophical and religious thought. It caused her to accept the experiences of life with a certain wisdom and fortitude. It was inevitable, perhaps, that she should try to plant seeds of this in my youthful imagination.

It was not long before I was formulating ambitions for the future, in a line which led along the path of an invalid. It seemed clear that I should have to spend the rest of my days leading a quiet life. This did not correspond with my nature, which was constantly calling for action far beyond my capacity to fulfil. It had been planned that I should prepare to become a lawyer, a career that would have been possible for me to undertake even under these circumstances.

As soon as I began rapidly to show a decided recovery under the hot Arizona desert sun, I sensed a deep inner frustration. Something was wrong within, and I did not yet know what it was.

2

In order to prepare myself for the coming term at school, I was permitted to go to our mining camp in the Dragoon Mountains, where I was to spend endless happy hours, working as well as playing. This range of hills is about fifteen miles out of town. The camp, however, was so far removed from all roads as to afford me complete privacy. The small hidden basin which was to be my summer home was situated at an elevation of about six thousand feet, in a section of the mountain, several miles in length, teeming with boulders of sandstone which would dwarf houses several stories high. Towering above my shack was Cochise Peak, some seven thousand feet up.

This part of the country was haunted with the spirit of romance. Formerly it had been the home of the Apache Indians, who had their hide-out in what is known as Cochise Stronghold. It probably seemed strange for a patient with an enlarged heart and the leakage of a couple of valves to be going into the mountains to recuperate. But having been raised in the higher altitudes, I actually began to feel better.

There was great joy for me in this retreat. From the moment I crossed the divide, leaving the outside world behind, I was in my mountain sanctuary, where the element of Time was completely removed. My illness had been severe enough and long enough wholly to cut me out of the race of external accomplishments. I could spend these timeless hours in contemplating and reading, and in digesting the thoughts gleaned from the books which I had brought with me. All these books were filled with Eastern wisdom; they were part of my mother's private library, which she had accumulated through the years. Their number was sufficient to cover almost every aspect of Eastern thought.

My mother's own life had been a quest for health

How My Interest in Yoga Began

and happiness, a quest in which she had left no stone unturned. And now her lifelong readings were being turned over to me.

I recall one of my first problems was that of diet, and in the years that followed I adhered strictly to vegetables, and even these were limited in number. On the other hand, having been a voracious eater, I still entertained dreams of sizzling porterhouse steaks. But these had to be banished as far as was possible from my thoughts. Not in a condition to put forth any physical exertion, I had the immediate problem of strengthening a body which had become emaciated from months of inactivity. The heart would not permit me to resume my old methods of physical training.

How to become strong again? All that was ultimately wanted was sufficient physical endurance to be able to meet the requirements of everyday work in an office. In the course of my early reading I recall a statement from Adams Beck's *Story of Philosophy*: " Infinite energy is at the disposal of any man if he knows how to get it. And this is a part of the science of Yoga." This offered me a line of hope. I immediately began to read everything I could uncover about this ancient spiritual science called Yoga ; for this was apparently the only thing that offered a way to me.

All the philosophical and religious books I had read stressed the fact that if I could hold the Right Thought anything I desired would be mine. The trouble was that it was impossible to hold the right thought long enough. I had learned from all previous training that it was one thing to be instructed, another to follow the instructions. The teacher could write out the rules of geometry or of any other subject on the board, but it was by my own efforts that it was possible for me to comprehend them and to be able to use them. All that the teacher could do was to guide me.

It was inevitable that I should arrive at only one possible conclusion, and this was that the spiritual aspect of the human body is no exception to this universal law of growth and development. The task was wholly mine. But how to make a beginning? The books dwelt upon the endless benefits to be derived from the practice of Yoga, but I could find nothing satisfactory on how to follow them. To be sure, I found no little stimulation in reading the lofty thoughts which the books contained, and I spent every spare moment in reading. For the time being, however, the question of practices had to be held in abeyance.

3

By the end of the summer I was ready for school, both in body and in heart. I had found an inner richness that I felt was to be mine until the end of my days. I had made up my mind to prepare myself for my work in life so that the economic aspect would be taken care of, the rest of my time to be devoted to study in this new world of thought that had been uncovered for me.

I searched far and wide for further reading material on Yoga. Moreover, I tried to get in touch with every person that I ever heard of who had been to India or knew anything about Indian teachings; for as time went on, the conviction grew that these teachings held the way for me. The exercises contained in the books which I had read were nothing more or less than variations of setting-up exercises that I had already learned and could do with the greatest ease. The breathing exercises seemed to hold the greater values, but somehow or other I could not successfully see the connection between the theory and the practice. I felt the need of a teacher. Actually, I did try even the breathing exercises, though in a rather haphazard sort of way. My heart condition being what it was, I had to be extremely cautious. Indeed, every book I picked up stressed the dangers of carrying on these practices without the aid of a teacher. How was such a teacher to be found, of all places, in Arizona? I had often read in my books of Eastern teachings that when a student was ready the teacher was sure to appear; moreover, that it was far more difficult to find the disciple than to find the teacher. This thought comforted me. At the same time, ignorant of what the future might hold, I devoted more and more of my spare time to the perfecting of such practices as were within my reach, without the assistance of a mentor.

Then, one day, out of a clear sky, I was summoned by one who had just arrived from India. He proved to be my first spiritual teacher or Guru.

For several generations there had always been some member of my family who had lived in India; so there was some tangible reason for what happened. My Guru knew all about me, and was fully aware of my late illness. I had long ago learned that the student was to hold a complete disregard for all matters of personal interest. So I did not question him concerning the mysteries of his appearance and of his knowledge of my existence. It was enough for me that he felt me worthy of his consideration. He was only passing through, and our meeting had to be brief. He having gotten in touch with me by wire, a time was set for a meeting.

As the time approached for his visit, my emotions were wrought up to a high pitch. My imagination, teeming with ideas and ideals, went off on a rampage. It was planned that I should see him after his evening meal at the place in which he was stopping. A visit which was to have lasted a couple of hours continued through the night; I left him at the break of dawn. He was a rather elderly man, of heavy stature and sensitive features, radiating spiritual strength. His eyes gleamed, and his voice rang like a bell. It was enough for me merely to sit in his presence and listen to the sounds issuing forth from his lips, sounds whose literal meaning I scarcely comprehended. Nevertheless they conveyed their own meaning to me, of a nature difficult here to define.

As might be expected, my first reaction was to give up the world and leave immediately for the hills, where I would spend my days in idyllic contemplation as a recluse. My Guru, however, pointed out to me that this was the way of the unenlightened, that such a course would be all in vain. He said: " All action without the guidance of intelligence is futile." I realized that his was a sane view, and for the first time I understood that I was put on my own, so to speak. He went on to tell me that the path of fulfilment was short, but that the path of preparation was long. In the years to follow, he added, I should not be impetuous about arriving, but should be ardent in my striving.

That I might have a picture of the scheme of things and understand the importance of the practice of Yoga by persons living in this era, he briefly outlined the teachings that had come down to him through the years of his discipleship, teachings which gave the student an idea of the world order.

In Indian philosophy, the universe in which we live has four ages in the same way that our earth has four seasons. Presumably, we are living in an age which is known as the Kali Yuga. One might think of it as the winter season. This age is recognized by its many manifestations, the chief of which are the actions of men. They are supposed to reveal much weakness at this time because of a depletion of vitality. Women are said to be coming into power. Everywhere there will be turmoil, struggle, chaos. People will show great restlessness, there will be much idle chatter, the hearts of men will be filled with pride, lust, ignorance of the real Truth. Men will be given over to gluttony, cruelty, selfishness, deceit, malice, depravity. Insanity will be in the ascendancy. There will be a great increase of litigation. Friendship will be on the wane. Men will crave luxuries, travel, gadding about. There will be great need of entertainment. Strictness in morals will be relaxed. There will be much hypocrisy. Deaths from diseases caused by Kaptha (phlegm) will be on the increase. There will be great droughts, famines, floods, hurricanes, earthquakes. Throughout the world nations will war against one another under the ægis of peace. People will be turning from their religious rites, which will have become nothing but empty form. Men will have lost sight of the Dharma (Moral Law) that was meant to pervade the form. This is an age in which men are " earth-bound."

4

There is only one path for liberation during this age, and that is to follow the path of Truth. The way to the Truth has been revealed for each age. During the first age, the Krita, or Satya Yuga, it was through the study of the Vedas, together with the observance of Dharma.

In the second age, the Treta Yuga, men found it more difficult to adhere to the strict rules of the Vedas. Hence, there came into being that body of literature known as the Smriti Scriptures, as the Laws of Manu and the Upanishads.

In the third age, the Dvapara Yuga, men gradually abandoned the rules and regulations prescribed in the Smritis; it was then that the literature known as the Puranas was revealed to them.

In the fourth and last age, the Kali Yuga, when the Dharma (the law of form and rule of right living) had all been completely destroyed, there was revealed for the liberation of men the Tantras,[1] which, it is believed, have the power to bestow Enjoyment as well as Liberation. The way given for liberation was through the practice of Yoga.

There is a great variation, however, in the method of Yoga. It undergoes changes with each age, and is different in its application to different individuals. Individuals have been classified in three general groups, according to their temperaments. Those of a pure physi-

[1] The *Tantras* were the encyclopædias of the knowledge of their time, for they dealt with nearly every subject, from the doctrine of the origin of the world to the laws which govern societies, and have always been considered as the repository of esoteric beliefs and practices, particularly those of the Spiritual Science, Yoga, the key to which has always been with the initiate and only passed on by word of mouth. Generically speaking, it is the term for the writings of various traditions which express the whole culture of a certain epoch in the ancient history of India.

cal nature come within the class known as Pashu. The mental class is known as Vira, while the last and highest group, possessing an extremely spiritual nature, belongs to the Divya class. It is clear that there can be an infinite blending and overlapping of these three groups. Hence, the worship and method of application will be different in each case. It is taught that not all men can worship alike, nor can all men realize the supreme experience by one and the same process. It is for this reason that different forms of worship and practice are prescribed by the Gurus, according to the particular temperament of each specific individual. The first requirement, then, is for the Guru to ascertain the peculiar qualifications of the disciple before he can attempt to initiate him.

5

Upon my insistence that I was ready to give up everything and devote the rest of my days to the indicated way of life, he pointed out that the four aims of man known as the Chaturvarga must all be fulfilled, and that only by taking one step at a time.

The first aim is known as Dharma, which demands that the individual first learn to live in accordance with Law. This is to be both Natural and Ethical, in harmony with the social order prevailing where one is living. Happiness is gained through obedience to Law; so one should first learn to adhere to the social law which is known to him. This will lay the groundwork for all further advance.

The second aim is known as Artha, which is the means by which the ultimate goal may be attained. In the world in which we are placed it is necessary that we look after all such material demands as food and shelter; it is essential that we attain some measure of material well-being if we are to have a chance to develop ourselves. Thus are we lifted above the animal kingdom, which lives only from day to day. By the accumulation of a modicum of wealth, which assures survival until some unknown point in the future, we are given

How My Interest in Yoga Began

sufficient leisure to devote a part of our energy to self-culture, instead, as in poverty, of dissipating it in a futile effort to survive. It matters little what one does as long as it conforms to the established law and order and is suited to his own nature, which functions in harmony with the Natural Law of Life. At all times one is reminded always to fulfil his own nature, for the laws of man are often in error. On the other hand, if one fails in some measure to follow the established order of things, he is rendered incapable of fulfilling his own nature. At all times it is necessary to use intelligence.

The third aim is known as Kama, which is desire and its fulfilment. This always means righteous desire, and it is here there is need of a teacher or guide. The parent is constantly telling the child that he may not carve his initials on the dining-room table. The child perhaps can see no reason for the restriction. But the day is surely coming when he will. The same principle may be applied to most men, who in the eyes of the enlightened are still children; I believe present-day psychologists confirm this view. It was at this point that the Guru told me that every one who has not yet renounced the world must seek happiness by meritorious desires and acts and the means by which they are achieved. In the beginning, people should cultivate all of these aims, for it is unworthy to follow only one. Each, in its own fashion, is a rung in the heavenward ladder of perfection. Severe condemnation is held for any one who is always engaged in ritual worship to the exclusion of his worldly affairs. As it is in our part of the world, there is a time and a place for everything.

The fourth and ultimate end of all sentient beings is known as Moksha or Liberation. There has been considerable philosophical discussion as to the nature of this state. The Tantras teach that it is the union of the personal self (or personal consciousness) with the universal self (or universal consciousness). This can be brought about by dispelling that condition of ignorance which supposes them to be different, and is achieved during this age through the practice of Yoga. From the Christian point of view, it might be considered as the attainment of their heaven; for the Buddhist it would be the reaching of Nirvana. Is it not the case that one and the other are talking about the same thing, but saying it in different ways? Let us not jump too quickly to conclusions.

The first three of these aims are known collectively as the Trivarga; they constitute the path of enjoyment, which is the way for every one in the beginning. The teachings assert that failure to traverse this path during one's lifetime reimposes the necessity of his doing it in his next earthly manifestation. When this obligation, however, has been carried out, the fortunate individual is then prepared to follow the ultimate aim, which is that of renunciation. The only place where man can gain Liberation is in this world; hence, his greatest blessing is the mere fact of his being alive. This world offers both, Enjoyment and Liberation; one must take each in its turn. This is the Divine Law.

It is in the order of things that the early part of one's life should be devoted to study and preparation, to the acquisition of knowledge; afterwards, the student should rigidly follow the discipline of his Guru. During this period, which may vary from a year to several years, the disciple must strictly observe the rules of Brahmachayya, one of which is to observe continence through the entire period of his initiations. At the end of this he is to return to the world and marry; he is to lead the life of a householder and accumulate wealth. During middle age he will devote himself to acts of charity and piety. When he has attained the age of fifty or thereabouts, having fulfilled the first three aims, he is to lay aside all worldly enjoyment and retire to follow the path of liberation. To-day man returns from the Stock Exchange, to *retire* and live the cultural life. In no circumstances must he leave his family in need. That is a sin.

6

As the light of a new day began to fill the room, my Guru once more reminded me that no harm could come to one during this age as long as he is purified by a knowledge of the Truth. It was taught that there was but One Truth, but that there were two ways of knowing it: the direct and indirect. It manifested itself in every aspect of nature, and through our senses it was possible for every man to know of it. Man had been endowed with the aspiration to go in the right direction, but because of his ignorance of the true purpose of the sense, he has become lost in his aspiration. It was in order to learn the Truth that the individual was told to follow the course of earthly enjoyments, for in this manner he would plant within himself the desire to perceive the truth directly. This could be accomplished only through Yoga. It is a way which calls for careful preliminaries, and demands strong faith. It is not the way for every one. The teaching is that man's mode of worship should always be according to his Adhikara, or competence, and that it is only if he worships within his Adhikara that he will enjoy the fruit of his worship. It is only thus that he will learn to know the Truth, and if he is well grounded in the Truth, he can evolve in this age.

In order to escape being harmed by this age, he is told to live free from malice, envy, hypocrisy, hatred, falsehood ; he must be frank and honest, devoted to the good of others. It is said no harm can come to him who keeps company with the Masters. It is important to strive for the highest levels of thought ; for ideas are the impelling motivating force of life. To desire perfection strongly enough, to have it in a real sense the guiding star in your life, is to be on the road to it.

7

Before I bade my Guru good-bye, he reminded me that the paramount purpose of my activities at this time was to prepare myself, in the first place, to be economically independent; for poverty was the worst of all evils. Poverty of the body, it was taught, led inevitably to poverty of the spirit. The most degrading poverty, however, was the poverty of the imagination; so I was at all times to keep in touch with the masters of the ages by reading all of the available philosophical literature. This was to include books on Western as well as Eastern thought.

Naturally, I was anxious to begin my Yoga practices immediately. He discouraged me from this, insisting that all things would come in their proper order. At this time my problem was to acquire the rudiments, lay the foundation. When I was ready, the rest would come. I was to maintain a standard of health, and develop as much physical strength as possible. Until I had gained a deeper understanding of their principles and had developed Yogic control over the body, I was to continue living in strict accordance with rules of health, adhering to my vegetable diet, and forgo acquiring the collegiate habit of smoking and indulgence in intoxicants.

He said it might be easy enough to condition the health of the body under Western methods. It was only when the time came for me to learn the techniques necessary for bodily purification and breath control that the Western training would be of no direct value. For these purposes he was going to give me two sets of exercises, one for the physical aspect of my body, the other for the mental; the latter would be very helpful in connection with my readings of Tantrik philosophy. He promised me a list of books dealing with this philosophy.

He suggested I do all of my reading while sitting in one of the many Asanas which are given in almost all books on Yoga. Asanas are merely the different postures which one assumes. I was not to be concerned about the reason for them, or to speculate on the nature of their benefits. It was enough for me to know that I could use them when the time arrived.

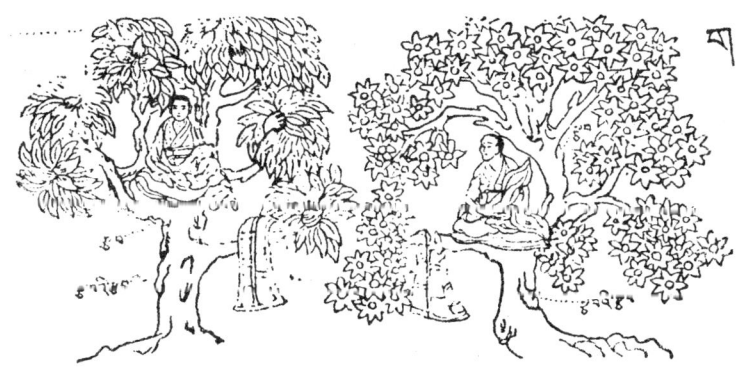

CHAPTER II

SOME PRELIMINARIES

I

THERE was one posture, said my Guru, which I should try to develop at this time. This was Padmasana, or the Lotus pose. This is considered to be the foremost of all Asanas, and it had to be learned if I expected to make any progress in the practice of Yoga. It is accomplished by sitting on the floor with the legs outstretched. Then the right leg is bent at the knee in such a manner that it is possible to fold it upon itself, placing the foot upon the left hip joint, and making the foot lie close to the root of the left thigh, or groin, with its sole upturned. The other leg is then to be similarly folded, the foot resting upon the right thigh, and as near the right groin as possible. The heels are to be set so as to be directly in front of the pubic bones, pressing upon the abdominal wall adjacent to it. The soles of the feet are to be trained so that eventually they will maintain their uppermost position. To relax and meditate in this position, the hands are to be placed on the heels with the palms turned upward, one hand resting in the palm of the other. If the left leg is uppermost, the left hand should rest in the right, and *vice versa*.

The Guru further advised me not to hurry, but to develop this Asana by slow degrees, until I could maintain it with comfort. It was of the greatest importance for future work that I should not attempt to maintain the position for more than an hour's duration without expert advice. At the time I could not see how I ever could do it for one hour, let alone longer.

2

My first exercise was to learn how to do the practice known as Uddiyana, or Inter-abdominal control. This calls for raising and lowering the viscera and diaphragm, which is attended by certain physiological effects. The debility of the muscles of the entire abdominal region causes stasis of its organs and parts; the healthy function of these organs is of the greatest importance in Yoga as well as in Yogic therapy. By means of Uddiyana the nerves and muscles of these organs are brought under the control of volition, and by the gentle shaking of the stomach and intestines these organs soon lose their lethargy and act with increased vigour, adding an abundance of health and strength to the disciple. My Guru would not go into the psychic benefits of this practice, for he was limiting his instructions to matters of bodily health, allowing me to discover the rest for myself as I developed the practice.

The technique for doing this exercise is to stand with the heels about a foot apart and with the body bent forward, the hands bent slightly and placed just above the knees. The body now is made to assume a semi-squatting posture, the spine describing a curve. The practice starts with a complete exhalation, which permits the diaphragm to rise to its highest level. When all the air is out, the muscles of the abdomen are vigorously contracted, the solar plexus being drawn well up under the ribs, the navel pressing as far as possible toward the spine. This contraction will naturally bring about a more forward bend to the trunk, which is what is desired. There is in this action a contraction of the two muscles of the back. These muscles being parallel and controlling the backbone, keeping it in place, are brought into play and made to exert an upward pull and inward push of the two muscles that run lengthwise on the abdomen from the junction of the ribs to the pelvis, producing a decided concave appearance. The diaphragm now occupies the highest possible position, having been sucked high up into the thoracic cavity. To help the muscular effort, one should stoop a little more and press on the knees with the hands, giving an upward push to the whole trunk. Having pulled all the muscles as far inward and upward toward the spine as possible, a sort of vomiting-like action is accomplished ; it consists in compressing the abdominal viscera and giving an added upward push. This upward and inward push is to be followed with repeated relaxations of the abdominal muscles. When the breath can no longer be suspended, all muscles are relaxed, the abdomen returning to its normal position ; the breath is then allowed to flow in.

In the beginning, the student should go very slowly. At no time is he to strain himself, go beyond his capacity ; an intensification of the exercises will come about naturally. At first, he should not do more of the contractions and relaxations on the suspension of breath than is comfortable. In other words, he should expel all the air in his lungs, and then contract and relax his abdominal muscles ten or fifteen times, depending upon how long he can hold his breath without any discomfort. Then he should stand up and breathe normally again before repeating the process.

Call that one round. The number of repetitions which the student will make of these rounds will depend upon the strength of his abdominal muscles. And he must not try them to the point of exhaustion. I was warned that regularity was absolutely essential. That is to say, when you decide you can do ten rounds of ten contractions each, making a total of a hundred vigorous contractions, it is compulsory that this standard be maintained regularly every day at the same hour over an extended period of time. I was advised to practise it every morning and every evening, and that the minimum number of times to do the exercise so as to derive benefit was 750, and the maximum 1500. He insisted that I should proceed very slowly and cautiously, keeping a close watch on every change that took place while practising. My ultimate goal was to do this 1500 times daily for a continuous period of six months.

3

This was to bring me to the ultimate development of Uddiyana, and then Nauli, which consists of gaining complete control over all the abdominal muscles, so that it will be possible to isolate the recti and roll them in any direction.

The exercise is accomplished by pulling the abdomen in as far as one can, as in Uddiyana, the side muscles being fully contracted; then the recti (the two erect muscles of the abdominal wall) are isolated and pushed forth. A forward thrust of the intestines is backed up by a downward and inward push of the muscles to the side of the straight muscles, and assisted by the posterior part of the diaphragm and the large triangular muscles of the lower thoracic vertebræ and the superficial triangular muscle upon the dorsal surface from behind. The thoracic muscles are also contracted, making the lungs press upon the diaphragm. This contracts under their pressure. The bowels are thus huddled up, bulging out under the isolated straight muscles of the abdomen. A sort of rolling motion is now performed, which gives the abdomen the appearance of an undulating surface of water. This is accomplished by contracting the left rectus, meanwhile relaxing all muscles of the right half of the abdominal muscles, letting them lie flat upon the belly. Now the rectus is rolled to the extreme left by making the contraction of the left side muscles more vigorous and the relaxation of the right side muscles more complete. When the rectus reaches the extreme left, the other muscles on this side are suddenly relaxed and the right rectus is made to stand out fully contracted on the extreme right border of the abdomen. The side muscles of the right are also stiffened. This movement gives the appearance of a wave that had in a moment transferred itself from the left to the right side. The right side muscles are now relaxed and the right rectus made to travel to the middle of the abdomen, when it is relaxed, transferring its contraction to the left rectus, which continues to be rolled to the extreme left with a wavelike relaxation following it.

The back muscles also play an important part in this exercise. The trunk being flexed upon the thighs, these back muscles remain contracted throughout the exercise, but the state of the contraction differs in the phenomena of the abdomen. When the rectus stands rolled off to the extreme left, the action of the back muscles is strongest on that side, and weakest on the right, resulting in the trunk being bent slightly to the left, while the front of the abdomen is turned toward the right side. As the rectus is being rolled to the middle, these muscles begin to relax, and by the time the rectus reaches the extreme right, the back muscles on the left side become tense in their action, and the right ones more powerfully contracted, flexing the trunk now to the right side, while the front of the abdomen turns to the left. Thus, there is a wavelike motion of the back muscles also. The diaphragm is likewise thrown into a wavelike motion.

It will be seen that every muscle that goes to form the abdominal cavity is alternately contracted and relaxed during the exercise of Nauli. The transverse colon is moved upward and downward through the largest space available in the abdomen. The rectum and descending colon may be shaken as well as the pelvic loop. No other exercise involves all the abdominal muscles and at the same time requires such vigorous contraction. This places Nauli at the top of all abdominal exercises. My Guru would not go into the benefits to be gained by this exercise other than the purely physical ones. He insisted, however, that I should develop it to the same point of efficiency as Uddiyana.

4

I was to supplement these exercises with the posture known as Sirshasana, otherwise known as the head stand. My Guru told me that I would realize great benefits from this, and that it was exceedingly important if I was to follow the prescribed path outlined for the disciple of Hatha Yoga, which is that form of Yoga which enables one to attain the inner union of the personal and universal consciousness by means of physical control. He would tell me nothing beyond giving me the assurance that for future mental development and control there was no practice equal to Sirshasana. He insisted that I would find greater physical and mental relaxation in this position than in any other, and that after I had developed it to a point where I could comfortably stand on my head for half an hour at a time, nothing could ever make me give it up. The period of half an hour, however, was scarcely a beginning, if I was ever to realize its maximum benefits. Indeed, it would be necessary, at some future time during my preparatory training, to develop it to the point of being able to remain on my head for three hours, and that I should maintain this practice for a period of at least a month, and preferably three months.

I immediately made a mental note of the time-consuming aspect of Yoga practice, but an inner determination told me that I would find the way. Again he warned me that I was at all times to proceed cautiously, adding that I should defeat my purpose if I tried to hurry. I was to think of it in the same way that one thought of a bed of flowers planted in the winter and expected to blossom in the spring. All one could do was to be patient while cultivating the ground. Nature never jumped a gap. At any rate, I realized that I was starting an entirely new rhythm of life, and that time was essential in order to perfect it. In the beginning, it was quite permissible for me to practise the exercise three times a day, thereby making the total time more easily

Some Preliminaries

attainable. Once I had developed the capacity to remain on my head for a straight period of three hours and could repeat this daily for an entire month, I could then lay aside the practice and feel that I had perfected it. This was the test, and what a test!

How was one to do it? There are no precise instructions. You are told, Just stand on your head! Do it in any fashion you can. If you find it difficult, here is the method generally recommended: First take a position on your hands and knees. Then interlocking your fingers, take such a position as to permit the forearms to rest on the floor. The interlocked fingers will now serve as a sort of bowl in which the head is placed. Now, the buttocks being raised, the lower end is lifted until it is perpendicular to the floor. In order to accomplish this in the easiest possible manner, put the weight of the trunk on the elbows and the head, which is being held firm by the interlocked fingers. Gradually the knees are to be raised and drawn in towards the elbows, with the toes still dragging on the floor. In this position the trunk is then thrown backward. Do this just enough to lift the toes off the floor until a perfect balance is effected. All movement should be done very smoothly, avoiding jerks to the body, for that is likely to upset everything and result in discouragement. After you have managed to maintain a balance in this position, lift the thighs slowly and bring them in line with the trunk.

I was told, "Take it easy." In the beginning I was to remain in this position for only a minute, making a mental note of everything that took place. For a week, or several weeks if necessary, I was to be content with this, repeating it at the same time thrice a day. Afterward, I could slowly begin to add seconds. I was to gauge my capacity by observing when the breathing began to get difficult and the perspiration began to flow. At this point I was to stop. Indeed, I was advised in all circumstances always to stay far within the safe limitations of my capacity, slowly increasing it with the

c

practice. The increase would come about of its own accord by regular practice over a period of time.

5

Daylight had come, and a new world had been revealed to me. It was impressed upon me by my Guru that Yoga had been devised by the ancient masters as a way for the people of this age to gain a direct understanding of the Truth. And again he stressed the fact that Padmasana, Uddiyana, Nauli, and Sirshasana were the first fundamentals for the practice of Yoga.

Having provided me with the techniques and the test for their perfection, the rest was wholly up to me. He would not advise how I should begin to develop them, or the order I should follow. It was, to use a colloquialism, a case of "take it or leave it." It was perhaps a part of my development that I should work it all out for myself.

Before I left him, he had something else to impart, and this he considered important. In the Orient, he said, it was customary for the disciple to perform many sacred rites before the practices were passed on to him; moreover, when initiated into the practices, he had to take the vow of "Secrecy."

This clearly held some meaning, a meaning which belonged to an old truth, but whose outward form changed with the times. The Guru reminded me of our own saying from the Bible: "Neither cast ye your pearls before the swine." In other words, it is wrong to give anything to the student until he is ready for it. He asked me if my parents had given me a 21-jewel watch as my first timepiece. Obviously, my answer was No; indeed I was still carrying the Ingersoll, which had long outworn its guarantee. He explained that in a fashion I had performed my sacred rites during my illness, for through that experience I had come to the realization that the way to eternal happiness was to be found within, and that in my quest of a method suited to me I had found that all hope lay in the practice of Yoga. Man might try to take short cuts and evade all form, but in the end he was bound to discover that there was no "short cut to Heaven." Nature withholds her secrets from us. It is still necessary either to follow the Path of Worship or the Path of Experience, which may be also called the Path of Suffering. We may see in this something of our own philosophy, which we seek to impart to the young student on finishing High School. He is told he can prepare for life in two ways: he can continue his training by going on to College, or he can learn in the School of Hard Knocks. This is the harder way.

In our own time forms have become empty; men have lost sight of the Law on which they have been constructed. Hence, it would be useless for me to take a Vow of Secrecy. It would be a purely superficial formality, without a real purpose. Nevertheless, I must try to maintain something of the spirit of such a vow. I was told that I must never tell any one about my practices. I should keep my every effort wholly to myself. How—it was up to me. Actually, he assured me, there was nothing mysterious about these practices. I could read about them in many books. Indeed—he said—there was nothing mysterious under the sun. Everything was working in accordance with the Divine Law. Happiness was harmony. This meant that the individual, by living in accord with the Law of which he is a part, will find happiness. It is this very Law that forbids revealing my efforts to others. Silence is Power.

He further explained that ideas were the motivating force of life, and that these are implanted in our consciousness by our actions and experiences. This must not be confused with mere factual information which we accumulate in the course of time. We are not moved to action until our thoughts find their way into our feelings; for no man is changed by mere logic. There are many ways of forcing thoughts into our feelings, and one of them is by intelligent suffering. The only way I could derive any benefit of ideas born in my illness was to direct their force into action. If I went around merely talking about it, it would not be long before they would be dissipated. We must never allow our anticipation to be greater than our realization, but this is what happens so often. It is only after I had perfected the practices and been fully initiated that I might talk about it to my heart's content. Not that I had to take a regular vow. It was that he wished to impress upon me that talking about a thing before you had done it caused a definite loss of energy, energy which should be used in carrying it out.

The time came for me to leave ; at six o'clock I had to open the restaurant where I was working in order to earn enough to enable me to go to school, for it was my parents' belief that one should always earn his way. As I shook hands with him in farewell, his last words were :

" Patience and perseverance are the key to salvation."

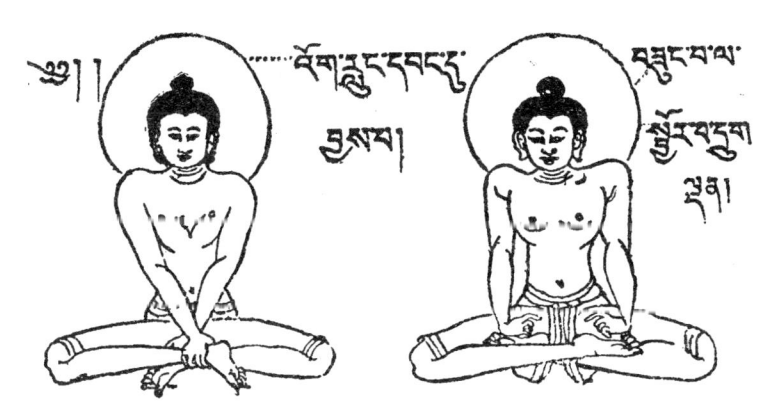

CHAPTER III

I MAKE A START

1

IT goes without saying that I encountered endless difficulties in my efforts to adhere to the practice programme given me by the Guru.

At school there was always a room-mate to cope with, to say nothing of the limited time at my disposal. I was working my way through school and trying to carry a full academic schedule. It could be seen that my problem was by no means easy, but it had to be solved, and eventually I did solve it.

The effort was not without its amusing side. I recall having almost been thrown out of a rooming house. Every month when the landlady came to collect the rent she would notice the grease-spot on the wall where my heels used to rub when I was standing on my head each day. Orders were promptly given to have it removed. But there it was again the following month. There seemed to be no reason under the sun to explain the mysterious recurrence of the grease-spot. After seven or eight months she finally, with a futile gesture, flung at me: "Heavens above! What on earth, my boy, do you do to dirty up the wall each month in the same place?" Flabbergasted, I sought desperately to find an excuse. I lamely suggested that there must be a hot-water pipe or something in the partition at that point which caused the wall to sweat. I doubt if my explanation satisfied her, but for the time being it quieted her. When I returned to school the following year she already had the room rented; so I sought elsewhere for a new victim.

I regained my health in a short while, and was able to spend the summer in the mountains working in the mines of my parents. By rising at five in the morning I had ample opportunity to adhere to the discipline I had given myself to maintain during the summer. There were also the evenings after work; I utilized these for practice and reading. As for the books recommended by my Guru, books I badly needed, it was a case of beg, borrow, and steal. I managed to get hold of many of the more important ones. It was always possible to read far into the night as I was not troubled with visitors or cinemas. These summers at the mine became the richest portion of my life.

With every successive year and the gradual perfection of the exercises, I began to enlarge my horizon of experience and contact by visiting the larger metropolitan areas, such as Los Angeles, San Francisco, Chicago, and finally New York. The greater part of my time was spent in combing the libraries, public and private. I tried to meet every one I had ever heard of who knew anything about these practices. I always presented myself as a complete novice, for I had been told by my Guru that I should never profess to know anything. This was for the reason that each individual might have a different aspect to offer, and only by keeping an open mind would it be possible for me to receive. At no time did I formulate any belief of my own. I was limiting myself to collecting philosophical precepts.

2

During these earlier years I maintained contact with the Guru by a steady correspondence. I wrote often, and no doubt at tiring length. Not an idea arose but that I would note it down. Never would he explain my problem. At best he would say that I was on the right path. It was not his method to teach me; rather it was to stimulate me to teach myself. He would merely call my attention to certain aspects of the problem in the light of what I had written. This would open a new door to me, only to find another closed door ahead. I shall never forget the weeks upon weeks of frustration, which would follow when I thought that I had a comprehension of the scheme of things as a whole, only to have him call my attention to the circumstance of the opposite philosophical way of life being just as feasible. All seemed very futile, for there appeared to be no answer. But then he would write that all things could be explained, and that eventually I would be given a Yantram (diagram or outline), which would embody every aspect of name and form manifest in Nature, making it possible for me to see how all the various phenomena of life fit into one cohesive, coherent whole. Every way of life would be the right way, in accordance with the Universal Law. But not all paths would lead one direct to the ultimate goal, though eventually all who would earnestly strive would find the Royal Highway to Heaven, the Path of Knowledge.

From time to time I would dwell in my letters on the inner experiences I was having in connection with my practices as I developed them. I was afraid I must have been prematurely drawing on my capacity. Thus, I was constantly upsetting my system while making tests as to the limits I could keep up in the practices and at the same time live what is for the American an active normal life. My teacher's answer was that I had to learn to use my head (not merely stand on it!), for common sense was the best teacher; it was for me to figure out what was wrong. In many instances the condition I complained of completely subsided before I received his answer, for he was far away and the mails were slow. If in the course of my reading I came across a practice I wanted to learn, my Guru's invariable answer was No. The time for that would come, he would say. Enthusiasm must be directed. The perfection of one practice was the perfection of all. I finally began to grasp his meaning. If I started jumping from one thing to another, I should eventually wind up with a smattering of all and knowledge of none. I should get nowhere.

3

After I had developed Uddiyana and Nauli to the maximum standard and had maintained it for over a period of six months, my Guru wrote me that I might begin to perfect the purification practices. He told me that these would be helpful in my efforts to hold the head-stand for three hours, which I was then struggling to do. At this time I reached the stage where half an hour on my head three times a day was the most resting and relaxing thing I could do. To do it for an hour was a struggle, but in the end I won out and thought that the rest should be easy. Once I tried to go the three-hour limit, I encountered difficulties. I began slowly by trying to do it for an hour and a half twice a day, but it became such an ordeal that I had to give up the attempt for a while. I got back-aches, stomach-aches, chest-aches, head-aches, and every imaginable kind of ache. The thing that most amazed people was my pulse-beat. When I was not running about, but spending the greater part of my time in reading and studying in one place, my respiration would get down to as low as three or four a minute, and my pulse would drop to as few as twelve. The doctors always wanted to put me to bed, especially those who knew about my previous condition. Actually, I had never felt better in my life. I had everything under such control that it was almost as if I had the power to turn my aches and pains on and off by the pressure of an electric-light button. Even as my teacher had foretold, there was an ever increasing appetite. The longer I managed to stand on my head, the more I could eat and not get fat. I could consume butter by the pound. My friends were impressed—and perplexed.

It was the greatest importance that one be clean, even

I Make a Start

to his veins, arteries, and nerves. In the first stage, one is to give his attention to all the processes which deal with the expelling of various secretions of the body. The bowels must be kept free from all feces and gases. The throat and stomach must be free from excess Kapha (phlegm). The acid of the stomach must be reduced to a minimum. The skin must perform its function perfectly; one should perspire a little each day.

The six processes of purification which Yoga has developed are called the Shatkarmas: Dhauti, Basti, Neti, Nauli, Trataka, and Kapalabhati. They are processes of elimination designed to clear away the impurities of the body and to correct any malformations or chronic diseases which may be due to impurities, or an imbalance of bodily vital principles. The six taken together are known as Sadhana, and he who practises them is called a Sadhaka.

The first, Dhauti, is thus divided: (1) internal washing; (2) cleansing the mouth; (3) cleansing the heart; (4) cleansing the rectum.

The second, Basti, has two sub-divisions: Wet and Dry, treatments of the anal sphinctures and colon.

The third, Neti, is a process of cleansing the head and its sinuses.

The fourth, Nauli, is a treatment or massage of the abdominal organs, already described.

The fifth, Trataka, is a practice for the eyes, with the aim of purifying and strengthening them.

The sixth, Kapalabhati, is a practice for cleansing the vascular system, designed to correct all disorders of Kapha (phlegm). Actually, it consists of three different practices: one is accomplished through breathing, the other two involve the use of water.

The daily cleaning of the ears, teeth and tongue is not to be omitted. In the process of cleaning the tongue by washing its root it is necessary to gain control over it and learn to swallow it. This is known as Khecari Mudra. I was to begin to learn how to do it; it was very important for my future work, though its precise purpose was withheld from me. The technique is simple enough. Every morning and evening after cleansing the root of the tongue with water by the aid of the second and third fingers, it is drawn out and gently milked and stretched in all directions in order to make it supple and flexible. In order to grasp it firmly, it is necessary in the beginning to use a piece of cloth. Silk is preferable. This is to be continued until it is possible to touch the tip of the nose with the tongue. The tongue is then turned back on itself in the effort to suck it back as far as possible into the throat. Eventually, one can swallow it with ease. As soon as the sensitive nerves in the affected region are accommodated to the touch, all unpleasant sensations will disappear. Six months should be spent in developing the practice. Ultimately, one will be able to go about with his tongue turned back all the time.

While perfecting this practice I suffered many embarrassing moments. As soon as you have swallowed the tongue, the mouth begins to fill up with saliva, which you are advised to swallow. I would be studying, or walking along the street, with a mouth full of saliva, when a friend would call out Hello. My usual reaction was a great gulp, which it was difficult to explain away, except by the remark that I had been day-dreaming. I was continually in a position where I had to make excuses for myself which never sounded quite plausible.

4

For the time being I concentrated on two of the six practices: Dhauti and Neti. My Guru conceded that it was not necessary to follow the Yoga methods of bodily purification when there was a Western method just as efficacious. Their methods had been developed centuries ago and were adapted to their way of living. The forms have undergone a constant change, and the new methods are just as good, if not more suitable to our present way of living. But how could I be sure? Hence,

I Make a Start

it was up to me first to go through the experience of a strict adherence to their rules; I had to learn all of their techniques. By mastering the methods of the East, I could readily readapt them to Western ways. Until I had thoroughly mastered them and been initiated into their esoteric purposes, I could scarcely pass judgment on their true meaning. What seemed to be a needless physical exercise might turn out to be of prime importance.

I was not to ask questions, I was to learn everything in due order. I have said this before, but it is something that cannot be stressed too often.

For the moment, however, instead of employing the process of Basti, I could utilize the enema for washing the colon; their method called for quite another technique, which I had yet to learn. As for the processes of Trataka and Kapalabhati, I could wait; these would come to be utilized in good time.

Dhauti is a process for cleansing and massaging the mucous membrane of the throat, œsophagus, and stomach with a cloth. It is recommended for removing excess phlegm, bile and other impurities of the stomach. Before practising Yoga one must always be free from phlegm, excess bile and gastric juices. For this purpose a cloth is used. It should be three or four inches in width and twenty-two and a half feet in length. A four-inch surgical gauze, cut to the proper length, is easily obtained and can serve the purpose.

The technique is simple. In the beginning, take a short dhauti, say two or three feet in length. After wetting it thoroughly, squeeze it out gently, so that it is moderately saturated with water. One end is then taken between the first and second fingers and inserted as far back into the throat as you can reach. It is left there to be swallowed in the same way that food is swallowed. A mock eating while gently inserting the dhauti bit by bit with the hand, coupled with the process of helping it with the tongue, will effectively send the cloth to the stomach. Sometimes a movement of the entire trunk, as though you were swallowing a large capsule, will speed up the process.

In the beginning, swallow only a few inches. After the throat has begun to accommodate itself, increase the length swallowed another foot or so. All soreness arising in the throat will soon pass away, so have no alarm. If the throat should persist in rejecting this intrusion, increase the saturation of the cloth. In the early stages the dhauti may be soaked in milk or sugar water if much difficulty is experienced in the swallowing of it. The more time that is spent in the beginning, the easier will it be to accomplish the swallowing of the dhauti. After the throat has been thoroughly adjusted to the cloth, it will be found that by a systematic daily practice you will, in about fifteen days, find yourself able to swallow the entire dhauti. It is really very simple.

If the throat is provoked to coughing, the eyes inflamed by tears, and the nose produces a discharge, I can only pass on the advice I received myself: "Do not despair." Simply postpone the attempt until the following morning. In no circumstance ever force matters, in no instance resort to rough treatment. Even in the most successful attempts, the throat, œsophagus, and stomach resent the irritation of the cloth, and there is a tendency to vomit it up. When this happens, close the mouth and rest a few minutes. After two or three spasms, the system will be ready to face another effort.

The withdrawal of the dhauti is simple enough, for it becomes very slippery with the mucus it absorbs. All that need be done is to give it a gentle pull. Sometimes the throat will lock on it. But shortly one will be able to open the throat and pull it out with both hands. The entire time spent in swallowing the dhauti, after one has perfected the process, will not be over ten minutes. In no instance should the dhauti be left in the stomach for a longer period than twenty-five minutes, for the stomach acts upon the cloth in the same manner that it acts upon food after the same length of time;

I Make a Start

there is a possibility of it passing through pyloric sphincter.

If by some almost impossible chance the entire cloth should slip into the stomach, there should be no cause for alarm. Employ a prompt emetic, and vomit it out. A saturated solution of salt water will be found to be very effective.

I was advised to carry out this practice every morning while I was working on the head-stand. This was for the purpose of removing the mucus that had collected during the night. It did not take long to master the process, but I must confess to many embarrassing moments. Again and again I let the door bell ring and ring. Sometimes, too, the 'phone would ring with a dogged persistence, due to the fact that the person ringing knew that I was invariably at home at this time. I let him imagine that I was in the tub. Or the person must have been perplexed at my voice, as I tried to talk to him over the 'phone with about fifteen feet of cloth within me and the rest dangling from my mouth. Privacy was an essential that one could not get around.

The other practice I perfected at this time was Neti, in order to cleanse the sinuses and region between the eyebrows, and to remove all the phlegm from the head. A thin thread is used in the beginning. You insert it into one of the nostrils, while holding the other end in your hand. By inhaling with some vigour, the thread will pass back into the throat, where it may be reached; it is then drawn out through the mouth. The thread is then slowly drawn back and forth through the nose and mouth. After a few minutes of this, the same operation is performed on the other nostril. In a short while it will be possible to use a larger string.

There is also the wet process of Neti; it consists of drawing water in through the nostrils and expelling it through the mouth. The process may be reversed by taking in a mouthful of water and expelling it through the nostrils. All these practices are extremely simple.

5

On finishing Law School I returned for a spell to my mountain retreat at the mine to take stock of myself. I began to ask myself: where was I going, and why? It was true, I had been told that I should find some way to become economically independent. It seemed to me that if I ever became enmeshed in the practice of law, there would never be any time left for my other studies; so I decided that I would follow the direction of philosophy. This would not only permit me to earn a living, but would allow me at the same time to give something of myself to the one subject that had become my very heart and soul. If I was ever to give instruction in these Eastern teachings in America, it would first be necessary that I fully acquaint myself with our own philosophical heritage. In the end, I hoped I would be in a position to interpret the East in the light of the West. As my final step in my preparation in the West, I registered at the Columbia University with the intention of taking a Ph.D. in the field of philosophy.

By this time I had perfected all of the physical training advised by my Guru on that unforgettable night of my life. I had found that everything he had told me was true, and I had gained an inner richness that could never be taken from me. I was fully convinced of that way of life being the right way for me. At the same time I had come to the realization of how much there was to learn. I knew I was still travelling in the Shadow of Truth rather than in its light. This could be attained only by going to India and being initiated. My Guru, with whom I had been carrying on so frequent and voluminous correspondence, was in India. He had insisted that I should not come to him until I had fully equipped myself with all the knowledge that was needful for me in the West. If I was to teach others, he said, it was imperative that I first make an intensive study of all the teachings of their way, for men could be helped only in the light of their own experiences. Not only was

I Make a Start

I to study philosophy as it is taught in academic circles, but I was to school myself in the teachings of all the religious sects that existed in my land. He again reminded me that Truth had an infinite number of manifestations, and that no sect, order, or creed had a divine prerogative on the Royal Road to Heaven. There were as many different ways as there were different kinds of people, but I should know of all ways in order to follow my own. This I tried to do.

The day of days came, when, having complied with the requirements given me by my Guru, I left for India to take up my studies under his direct guidance. It seemed like a dream coming true.

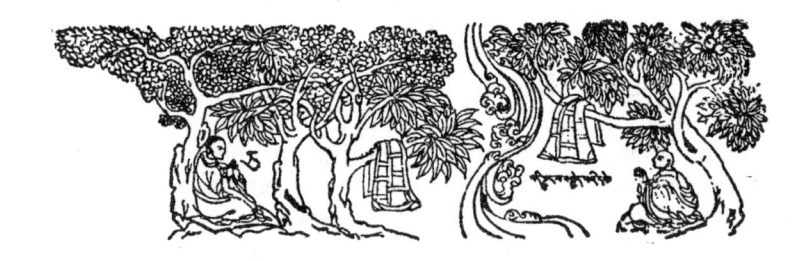

CHAPTER IV

I GO TO INDIA, THE HOME OF YOGA

I

INDIA has been fittingly described as "a land that nobody knows. One million eight hundred square miles of it, teeming with shrines and squalor, fantasy and filth, rajas and ruin; a kaleidoscope of pageantry and poverty, holiness and hate, dust, diamonds, and festering death, but always a land of mystery."

On landing in Calcutta I was so excited I couldn't bother about the details of checking my luggage, and I still don't know how my trunks ever reached the hotel. I recall stepping into an open gharry (Indian taxi-cab), driven by a heavily bearded Sikh who was attired in a sweaty khaki shirt, and as I turned my head on leaving the pier I saw my trunks following on the heads of a couple of extremely frail-looking coolies.

Reservations had been made at a hotel, where the clerks greeted me as though I were an old patron. The moment I reached my room I stripped myself to the skin and started the large fan going full blast. Even so, I was sweating as if I were working with a pick and shovel under the Arizona desert sun. After consuming a couple of lemon squashes I dashed off a letter to my teacher, notifying him of my arrival. It had been some time since I last received a message from him, as I had been too much on the move to write. I had arrived at the end of the monsoon, and I was told that many of the railways had been wholly washed away. This meant that

I Go to India, the Home of Yoga

there might be a considerable delay before I could receive an answer.

After I had made several trips a day to my letter box for almost two weeks, the message which I had been expecting finally arrived. I didn't recognize it at first, for it came from the head of the family with whom my teacher had resided for some years. In India it is customary for a holy man to be taken care of by a rich family, whose members may be called his spiritual patrons. The first page was one long, fervent greeting, welcoming me to India. After that, the writer went on to say that my teacher was away at the moment, and that one of the family would come to town to see me. I was, emotionally, in a ferment of anticipation.

On the following day the eldest son of the family arrived. He was just my age. I had already heard much about him. For some years past it had been planned that when I came to India the two of us would begin the study of Sanskrit under the guidance of his learned father. The meeting was very casual. There was prompt recognition on both sides, as we had previously exchanged photographs. We plunged into conversation, and were so deep in it that several hours passed before I thought to ask when my Guru would arrive. He said that was what he had come to talk to me about. Indeed —I was hardly prepared for the shock—my Guru had passed away only a few days before my arrival!

I did not dare reveal my inner feelings to my visitor. Actually, I did not fully grasp the full meaning of my loss until I was left alone, when I was overcome by a sense of deep frustration. Where could I turn for guidance? I was emotionally very much wrought up. At that moment I realized how deep was the gap between learning philosophy and being philosophical over the tragedies of life. For me, surely, at this time my Guru's death seemed like a tragedy; though for these holy men death was as much a part of life as was birth. It gave the spirit of man an opportunity to revitalize itself, and to manifest itself anew in another form.

D

2

On the following day I had a visit from the young man's father, a fine scholar who came of a family that had produced great scholars for generations. He well understood my loss, which was also his loss. Apparently they had discussed me for years, and my letters, revealing the gradual maturation of myself, were familiar to him. This knowledge of me was greatly to my advantage, for the sincere persons of that land do not readily reveal themselves to strangers in the early days of their acquaintance. So many have come and gone, making light of their cherished beliefs. Once this gap of uncertainty has been bridged, they will spare no time or effort in doing all that is within their power to enable the erstwhile stranger to continue his quest, and indeed will consider it their duty to do so.

My visitor suggested that I promptly meet a certain Tantrik, who would act as the mentor in my ensuing studies. No sooner said than done. We called a gharry and left the hotel in search of this Tantrik, who was not known to my companion personally. We drove through the characteristic maze of a large Indian city, first stopping at a relative's house, some miles from my friend's home. There we were directed to the house of a friend, who told us to consult yet another friend. At last we found ourselves outside a large compound surrounded by a high wall, whose entrance was closed by a huge iron gate.

After some explanation the gatekeeper sent another servant to the master of the house to report the arrival of strangers. Once admitted within the walls of the compound, we hurried on to the house, a two-story red-brick structure. A servant conducted us to our host's study on the second floor, where refreshments were at once ordered for us. After introducing himself and me, my friend proceeded to explain the reason for this rather informal intrusion. A cordial relationship was promptly established. It turned out that our host was a

I Go to India, the Home of Yoga

very intimate friend of the Tantrik whom we desired to meet.

As the day was drawing to a close, we begged to be allowed to take leave in order, without delay, to pay an immediate visit to the Tantrik, to whom we now had an introduction. On arrival, we were ushered into the private sanctum of the man we had been seeking. My friend explained the object of our visit; then, as the hour was late, he left us.

I remained a long time with the Tantrik after my friend had departed. Even on first meeting I had the feeling that in this man was the real source to all that I had so long sought. A large man, with a very kindly face, and with the light of intelligence and understanding illuming all his features, he seemed like a father to me. He was leaving in a couple of days for a short spell away from the city heat in his jungle retreat, and asked if I could join him. The monsoon having just passed, it was growing very hot, so the opportunity for this stay in the more wooded and cooler regions promised a welcome change. Incidentally, my host suggested that it would give us an interlude of leisure, which would permit us to know each other better.

The words of my Guru came back to me: "When you are ready, a teacher will appear."

3

We had constant talks upon all subjects, and particularly upon things Tantrik. Our talks keyed me up to great expectancy. I felt quickened, my dream seemed on the verge of realization.

During the first days he apparently sought to determine the measure of my knowledge and comprehension of the principles which I had been studying alone. It was useless, he said, to proceed with Yoga practices without understanding. So we took up a rather brief outline of the subject. He pointed out that Yoga is activity scientifically applied. By means of its practices, diseases of the body are destroyed, and health and happiness established. It will develop the intelligence and bring one to a True Knowledge of Self. He said that it could be applied to every aspect of life. Yoga is also defined as mental abstraction, as silent prayer, as the union of the mind and soul, as the art of suspending the circulation, as that which suspends the outer expression of the world of feeling, as dexterity in performing any kind of action (whether spiritual, mental, or physical), thereby obtaining the right results, as a method, a process, of body culture and mind control, as a system of applied psychology more highly developed than any known to Occidental sciences, as a science of human culture in the highest sense of the word.

The word Yoga itself is said to have seventeen meanings:

1. Union, or methods of union.
2. Any outside thing united to any other outside thing.
3. To mix one thing with another, as sugar with water.
4. To unite cause with effect, as sparks with fire.
5. The method of properly decorating, keeping things in their proper places.
6. Some symbolized word which reveals an internal meaning, as a cable code, proverb, or aphorism; these are also called Yoga.
7. To hide one thing and to try to show another, signifying a thing without telling about it, as a hint, or as a magician would do.
8. Different significances of words, which vary according to different minds.
9. Physical exercise.
10. Proper composition of language to convey description.
11. Any sort of skill or dexterity.
12. Methods to protect what one possesses, materially, mentally, and spiritually.
13. To find means for acquiring things by deep contemplation, as the solution of a problem in mathematics

I Go to India, the Home of Yoga

or in engineering, or the unveiling of a plot as in a problem story.

14. Conversion of one substance into another, such as the creation of something new out of a known substance, as in chemistry.

15. To unite two souls for any purpose.

16. To produce a current of thought for any specific attainment, to take any specific object or concept and make the mind follow it to the exclusion of all else.

17. To suspend all mental activity, to concentrate the heart upon one particular thing.

From this variety of definitions it is possible to grasp something of the breadth and scope of Yoga. Clearly, it appertains to all of life in its infinitude of manifestations. It is a science devised for man and his functions. No matter where he may walk or what he might do, it will guide him to the path of liberation. The best proof of the practical nature of Yoga is that every system of religion and philosophy in India has recognized Yoga as the most scientific means of realizing truth. Men of great mental powers and courage in India, Tibet, and China have invariably been the product of the teachings and practice of Yoga. It is taught that Buddha, Confucius, Milarepa of Tibet, Krishna, and even our own Jesus Christ, had received their divine enlightenment in this way.

Yoga teaches the existence of a subtle force in man, and how this force may be controlled and made to function so that man may gain his absolute freedom. The practice of Yoga keeps the mind firm in joy and suffering. It gives one foresight in speech, in action, and in freedom, saving him from all distress and apprehensions of the mind. It is the shortest and most direct path to the knowledge of all things.

Its first aim is the achievement of detachment from the world. This does not mean isolation from it. Rather it teaches one how to be in the world, yet not of it. Its second aim is to gain restraint over the mind and its creations. This purifies the manifesting consciousness. By its practice the mind automatically becomes filled with high aspirations, and acquires great spiritual power even while all the unhappy tendencies die out. Its third aim is the attainment of the condition of eternal Samadhi, which is complete union, the positive identification of the Soul with its parent, of which man is but a part. This is the ultimate goal of all Yoga.

As by knowledge and practice of the alphabets all languages can be learned, so by the practice of Yoga, which is the alphabet of life, one can attain by degrees a knowledge of Truth. As gold can be separated from impurities by methods of chemistry, so can Truth be divorced from error by methods of Yoga. It gives the devotee a tangible knowledge of the future and the unseen. It makes men capable of appreciating the life around them and gives them the power to make that life worth appreciating, regardless of the circumstances and the stress of the times in which they must live. For the Yogi, happiness is eternal. What the intellectual, moral, and spiritual man hopes for, whatever he loves, wishes, or wills, is to be found in this enchanted castle of Yoga. This union, or Yoga, when accomplished by the individual, must enhance his sensibilities and his powers; and a far-reaching knowledge of the secrets of Nature is his.

The Yogi comes to live above, or apart, from material matters, and only enters into such things in his daily life as he is bound by custom and the need of them for the maintenance of his body. He is disdainful of this material world, because it is a source of delusion and enslavement.

4

Man's paramount aim, according to Yoga philosophy, should be that of freeing himself from three kinds of pain:

1. That arising from his own infirmities and wrong conduct, such as disease.

I Go to India, the Home of Yoga

2. That arising from his relationship with other living things, such as wild animals and persons who try to take advantage of others.

3. That arising from his relationship with external nature, such as the elements and other abstract and subtle powers.

The systematic study of Yoga has been in a state of decay these past several hundred years because of the idleness, ignorance, and unscrupulousness of its followers. The canker of laziness, selfishness, vanity, and delusion commenced its work of destruction at the beginning of the Kali Yoga. Corrupted rites, false ideas, and dogmatic tenets led men to corruption. The Yogis were finally compelled to retire to secret abodes. Only remnants of true Yoga are accessible to-day to the seeker. Even in India, the home of Yoga, supreme ignorance prevails about Yoga in general, a criticism which does not exclude the educated circles.

Yoga has been one of the most neglected portions of East Indian teachings. This is largely due to the tremendous advance of material sciences. Man has been so predominantly devoted to material and physical pursuits, and to purely experimental or empirical science, which demands the use of the faculties of observation, that he has sacrificed in the process the higher faculties of reflection, imagination, and abstraction, which alone can serve him in ultimate things and provide a true perspective on that part of human existence which alone matters.

There is no question that the prevailing material philosophy has failed to achieve its object, i.e., the increase of the sum total of human happiness; hence, it stands self-condemned. It tends to generate an insatiable hunger. It never leads to contentment, it develops in man a cold, calculating greediness. It cannot be said that it has made a single soul happy; it has surely cast a shroud of gloom and doubt over the spiritual attributes of man.

These worldly philosophies are like medicine. They give temporary relief from an ever-recurring pain, while true philosophy gives eternal peace and happiness. True wisdom does not consist in increasing our wants, but in reducing our needs. This comes about only as we retire within. What men consider to be pleasure is but a modified form of grief; and it is transitory. Its absence brings pain. The more we enjoy, the more we are apt to become miserable, for with the increment of the objects of pleasure, our desires and wants also increase. And, in any event, sooner or later, there comes the approach of old age, and the end of such enjoyment. Of what avail, then, are wealth and the pleasure that wealth gives?

The higher man seeks what he wants within himself, while the ordinary man has no aim other than to discover and enjoy things on his way through life. The material things of the world can be taken away from him, but nothing can take from the higher man the understanding, or Truth, that he has gained through the science of Yoga. And it was this precious secret that I had come to India to learn.

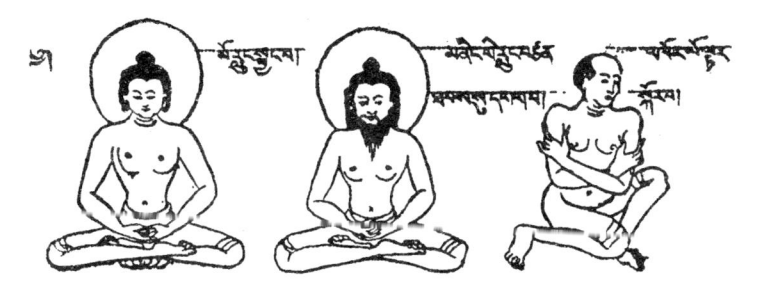

CHAPTER V

THE MEANING OF YOGA

I

"As water continually exudes from a broken vessel, so our period of life is being constantly shortened; yet death is as much a portion of life as night is of day." Death and Life are only two aspects of nature. One works from the outside and tends to keep the individual centres apart; the other works from the inside, in the effort to perpetuate itself. The outer force which pulls us apart is Death; the inner force that keeps our units of experience together is Life. Together they form the process of becoming, of evolving.

Before we can fully understand man, we shall have to examine the force which sustain him and make him what he is. These finer, more abstract energies are always invisible. The physical aspects of the body can be seen through its own instrumentality, but the abstract energies of the body require the power of spiritual perception. Yoga is the method by which this is possible. In order to attain this end, the first object is to conquer the six enemies:

1. Desire for sexual and other enjoyments.
2. The urge to injure others.
3. The appetite for wealth and the like.
4. Ignorance of the real.
5. Pride of birth, wealth, learning, etc.
6. Envy.

These are to be conquered by the "eight limbs" of Yoga, according to the teachings of Raja Yoga, which is the ultimate form of all Yoga. They are divided into the outer and the inner practices, the outer consisting of the aspect of mentally controlling the different energies of the body:

1. Yama, control.
2. Niyama, regulation.
3. Asana, posture.
4. Pranayama, breathing practices.
5. Pratyahara, restraint, withdrawal.

The inner processes which culminate in attaining spiritual perception are:

6. Dharana, concentration.
7. Dhyana, meditation.
8. Samadhi, communion or a state of superconsciousness.

Since these "eight limbs" are so fundamental for anyone preparing to practise Yoga, it would be advisable to present a brief outline of the principles behind these steps, as they were given to me. This should enable each student to gauge for himself as to how the different principles may be applicable to him in his present environment.

Yama and Niyama provide the mental discipline, the preliminary requisite to all Yogic culture. They aim to liberate the mind from strong emotions and to enable the individual to develop the contentment so essential to a perfectly balanced mind. Yama calls for discipline to restrain the evil tendencies to which all flesh is heir. Under this head are included the highest moral maxims of a religious and ethical nature. It provides for:

1. Disinclination to injure others, absence of all violence toward all living creatures, absence of anger toward an aggressor, imperturbability, compassion to all life.

2. Avoidance of untruth, the practice of universal innocence, of humility.

The Meaning of Yoga

3. Disinclination to steal.
4. Disinclination to sexual enjoyment.
5. Non-coveting, non-desire of things belonging to others, disinterestedness, non-acceptance of gifts.
6. Restriction of food to essential needs for the preservation of the body.
7. Everlasting purity

Niyama provides discipline in the field of moral attributes, strength of character, forbearance, patience while suffering injuries sent by the fates, non-complaint, retention of calm in circumstances tending to provoke vexation and irritation. It calls for penance, contentment, self-denial, purification of one's thoughts, belief in the continuity of Jiva (soul) leading to the practice of Dharma (religious merit), listening to religious and philosophical teachings, aversion to low and wicked practices, discrimination, and recitation of Mantras (mystic sounds) with concentration—in the manner enjoined by the Guru. One must give charity according to one's means, discharge all debts due to one's teacher or higher mentors through whom one has profited. One must also worship the one Supreme source of wisdom and power, and give devotion to one's own form of the Supreme Being adopted by the Sadhaka. Cleanliness, likewise, comes under this division. The utmost care in attending to the body and apparel is enjoined upon one. Yama and Niyama mean moderation in every habit, and a living faith in the Supreme.

Frugality of diet is said to be the most essential of the Yamas, while non-injury is the greatest of the Niyamas. Only those whose minds are disturbed by anger, lust and like evil propensities, and prone to physical and mental uncleanliness, are enjoined to practise Yama and Niyama. Strict observance of these rules brings its own rewards. A man free from these and other vices is qualified for Yoga without preliminary preparation.

It is now clear why my Tantrik friend was devoting so much time to me. He was not going to put me in contact with a new Guru until he was certain that I was fully prepared. This could be determined only through days of intimate association. All this time I was asking questions, and these questions would reveal to him indirectly the growth of my inner self.

2

Then comes Asana. This means posture, or right position. The fundamental postures are four:

1. Padmasana.
2. Siddhasana.
3. Swastikasana.
4. Vajrasana.

I will later, in their proper sequence, speak of these in detail.

Pranayama deals with the specific methods of working the breath, thereby restraining the mind.

Pratyahara is nerve control. It is the accommodation of the senses to the nature of the mind, inducing the absence of concernment with the object of each respective sense. The withdrawal of the sense functions will produce abstraction, which gives calm and courage, and makes the mind introspective by turning it back upon itself. Pratyahara is of five kinds:

1. The forcible withdrawing of the sense from attractions of the objects of sense.
2. Contemplation of all that one sees as the Self (Atma).
3. Making the mind introspective and one-pointed.
4. Renouncing all fruits of action, working for the joy of accomplishment.
5. Restraining all outward emotions.

The fruit of Pratyahara is the overcoming of the objective world by the subjective, and the exaltation of the imagination to so high a pitch as to cause all of its images to stand forth vividly on the canvas of objectivity. Pratyahara always stands at the gate leading from the outer to the inner world; without it, the withdrawal of

The Meaning of Yoga

the senses from their objects is impossible. It is the preparatory process to Dharana.

Dharana is attention, mind control, the first step in preventing the mind from wandering about at large, and in directing it to a single point. It is the binding of the mind to one place. It is the power to hold an idea in mind for the purpose of meditation.

Dhyana is the becoming one with the idea. The process being eliminated, the subject is merged in the object. In this process the consciousness is fixed upon a single object without a break. There are four Dhyanas:

1. A state of joy and gladness born of seclusion that is full of investigation and reflection.
2. That born of deep tranquillity without investigation and reflection.
3. Destruction of passion.
4. Pure equanimity, making an end of sorrow.

Samadhi is that ultimate bliss, isolation, superconsciousness, emancipation, or ecstasy, that is the craving of every heart. It has many degrees, and we have all tasted of some aspect of it at one time or another during our lives. There are two methods to Samadhi. One is to detach oneself from everything that one sees, hears, feels, etc., to retire within, to deny all things. In short, we have complete self-abnegation here. The second method is the constant practice of Yoga. The signs of Samadhi are the negation of all positive manifestations of life, and the complete enthralment or subjugation of all objective thoughts. The object is to attain that state in which a man will be the same in want as in prosperity, and be free from lust, fear, and anger. He will be the same in hatred as in love, with enemies as with friends, and wholly unaffected by honour or dishonour.

The great father of Yoga, Patanjali, gives us the following primary distractions as obstacles in the effort to attain this supreme state of consciousness:

(1) Sickness; (2) Languor; (3) Doubt; (4) Careless-

ness; (5) Laziness; (6) Addiction to objects of the senses; (7) Erroneous perception; (8) Failure to obtain any measure of abstraction; (9) Instability when attained.

The secondary distractions are:

(10) Grief; (11) Distress; (12) Trembling; (13) Sighing.

My Tantrik friend said that possibly the greatest of all hindrances to the practice of Yoga were such sensual pleasures as the enjoyment of sex, dancing, music, luxurious bedding, beautiful cosy corners, fine clothing, the eating of rich food and meats, travelling in excessive comfort, voluptuous habits, frequent feeding of guests, pleasure and reputation-seeking, the enjoyment of wealth, and money-hoarding. Other hindrances were: ambition (even in religious matters), bad company, false and vain controversies, cruel, harsh speech, lying, promiscuous visiting, gregariousness. The mind dominated by sensation is doomed to fail in any attempt at self-mastery. It is wrong to be continually observing vows, practising silence and fasting, oppressing the body, making pilgrimages to places of worship, and carrying on useless contemplation, and not giving satisfaction to one's Guru.

3

Now everything was beginning to assume a new depth of meaning, now I began to see how these practices might be applied to all of us in the West. I could see the rules observed during my training period assuming a significance. Behind them there was something more than rules for pure physical culture. Social customs, which hitherto had seemed useless and aimless, began to show some semblance of purpose. Principles of applied psychology were shaping into the scheme of things. One in all, everything was slowly finding its way into one great cohesive whole. I could now understand the saying that learning is the perception of differences, while wisdom is the perception of similarities.

The Meaning of Yoga

A definite time of day was set aside for our talks, for my Tantrik friend adhered to a rigid discipline. He was always up by four for his early morning meditations. I had not yet left my American habits far enough behind to be able to rise with comfort at that early hour, so I did not get my Chota Harzi (early morning tea) until five. I was still filling the rôle of student rather than of practitioner. My early morning hours were mostly spent in reading and reflection, and I spent many hours in doing Yogic practices I had learned in America. I would always begin the day with a few rounds of Uddiyana—this just before the tea came.

As soon as I was fully awake, I would go for a stroll through the jungle. There was always a gentle breeze in the early morning, and the stir of nature awoke a response in me and quickened all my faculties. The days in India are quite unbearable, but then the loveliness of dawn is not to be paralleled anywhere. These ecstatic dawns stimulated the creative spirit and helped me to find the answers to problems of the day before. About seven-thirty I would return to my small adobe room with its thatched roof, which helped to keep it very cool under the sweltering noonday sun. The servants always had my tub ready, so that I was sure to appear for breakfast on time.

This was usually a leisurely hour, and sometimes it was prolonged until ten o'clock. By eight o'clock, when we sat down on the floor to our morning meal, my host had already finished what was equivalent to half a day's work. Little wonder that India has produced so many scholars, for they waste very little time. This portion of the day was crowded with discussion, mostly touching on philosophy. We would always start with some minor incident of experience, and eventually it would lead us to discuss the philosophical principle behind it. By this method I was gradually learning how everything under the sun was united in the Supreme, and that a knowledge of the principles of philosophy enabled one to find a synthesis for a variety of facts and experience.

Debatable points were postponed for discussion at teatime, as he was busy for the rest of the morning. After lunch we would have our "siesta." I read much during this period. The rest of the day and evening was usually devoted to conversation, sometimes lasting far into the night.

I think I asked many absurd questions, sometimes because I didn't know any better, sometimes on purpose, for I was trying to see everything in the light of present-day Western thought. It was my desire to reconcile—at least in my own mind—the East and the West. So often I had heard that it was impossible for the Westerner to practise Yoga, as if the Easterner were some special sort of animal, endowed with different gifts. I had come to the reasonable conclusion that rules laid down for man in the East might work anywhere. The mere crossing of an ocean did not change the human constitution or rearrange the atoms of the human body. Only the outward forms were different, the man within remained the same. To be sure, I carried my own little bag of prejudices that had been handed down to me by my own culture which it was impossible for me to throw off hastily. Despite it, something within me was at all times in complete accord with the tenets of Yoga. In any event, I kept my eyes open to discover any form among us that manifested the same principle. Only thus had I any hope of discerning the philosophical scheme of things. Only thus might I readapt new forms to Eternal Truths. For it is only the form that changes, never Truth.

4

Certain erroneous ideas prevail about the practice of Yoga. Among them is the notion that its disciples take a pronounced delight in knowledge *per se*, and in the development of the body *per se*. Others are that study and practice are employed for the subjugation of the senses, that one counts on awakening Kundalini (psychic energy) by certain physical practices alone, that devotion

The Meaning of Yoga

to the paths of knowledge will have the desired effect on the Nadis (nerves) and senses (subtle and gross), and that Samadhi (trance) can be induced at once by taking certain chemical essences, or by the eating of certain foods. It is true that Opium, Bhang, Charas, Ganju, and a special kind of wine under skilled administration are used by some who are advanced in Yoga practices to induce a rapid state of mental abstraction, but this cannot be done by one possessed of an impure body and improperly or insufficiently trained in Yoga.

Westerners seem to have the idea that it is impossible to practice Yoga while leading a domestic life. I asked my friend to clear up this point. His answer was that wealth and family environment were by no means an obstacle to Yoga if the person properly performed his Yoga duties. Yoga was not for the ascetic alone. It was the common heritage of all, the rich, the poor, the learned, and the unlearned. Men of mild temperament, to be sure, would not be attracted to Yoga practices. Such persons should seek advancement along the path of virtue and devotion. As for marriage, far from being a hindrance, it should actually facilitate one's development. It is not to be gainsaid that the first and foremost temptation the student meets comes from his passions, and the strongest of these is sexual desire. To yield to this desire in moderation, however, is an essential condition in success.

It is true that those who practise the vow of Brahmacharya (Sanskrit for celibacy) believe that sexual abstinence is a positive necessity to all spiritual culture, and that Yoga should not tolerate any condition but that of celibacy. Actually, this is not an absolute injunction in Yoga, but Chastity is. Moderation is an incontrovertible precept in all things related to Yoga. Some of our most spiritual types of men have been heads of families, and some of the foremost Yogis have been married men with families, and even with kingdoms to look after. The Kularnava Tantra says: " By what men fall, by that they rise."

E

In some instances, sexual indulgence is detrimental, even injurious to the goal sought. Once, however, the practice of Yoga has been accomplished and the goal reached, there is no rule to bind one to celibacy. Conserved sex energy gives power to develop the suspension of breath, and the more one is able to preserve the essence of sex, the more light there is to be seen in the heart.

In the higher forms of Yoga practice there is greater conservation of energy and nerve force. Here there is no place for sexual pleasure, the practitioner's pleasures having been elevated to a higher sphere. Sexual pleasure is not abandoned because of its harmful effects, but simply because it has disappeared from the realm of desire, in the same way that the game of marbles, the doll, the playhouse, and all other childish recreations have disappeared from the realm of desire of the grown-up. In these stages of Yoga, the practices themselves tend to sublimate sexual forces and to transmute them into higher activities. Such a condition, however, does not prevail in normal Yoga experience, and the man practising Yoga is scarcely called upon to go to extremes in this matter of sex.

5

Philosophical curiosity is the first step in the mental ascent towards Yoga. This is why the teacher studies his pupil so long before he allows him to do any of the practices. The process of the birth of philosophical curiosity is not unlike that of the birth of desire. The impulse of desire comes from the external world, while that of philosophical curiosity comes directly through the mind. The strength of the latter depends upon the mind's power of reflection, and as this power is relatively weaker at the beginning than that of desire feeding on external stimuli, the mind must be encouraged and trained to take stock of itself ; it must be taught to withdraw from the outer world in order that it can concentrate on spiritual things, not perceptible to the senses.

The mind truly begins to function when it begins to ask questions about itself and stops drifting hither and thither in the blind way it has before attaining a measure of discipline.

Self training calls for selective, intensive work of mind and body. What man has learned to control becomes part and parcel of his emotional life, which is then really his own.

To my question, " How does one begin, and what are the stages of development in the practice of Yoga? " my Tantrik friend said that the devotee, first of all, was required to learn how to sit, since this was an art which gave him control over his body and all its parts. The postures are calculated directly to hold the physical forces in balance and indirectly to develop mental and spiritual powers. In the second stage he will take up the practices of particular breathing exercises which will enable him to steady the mind so that it can be centred on one worthy object and lose itself. After he has mastered these practices, he will find that in the third stage he will be able to exercise such restraint over his senses that it will be possible for him to realize more vividly the object he holds in his mind. In the fourth stage he will be able to hold the object of his worship in his mind for contemplation. In the fifth, when the mind is able to hold its object for some length of time, he is able to realize it undisturbed by Self and his surroundings. After the perfection of this stage he will come to the sixth, which is accomplished when the mind can unite with the Deity. This stage represents the highest effort of the finite mind, and it comes to pass only when a pure and complete absorption of the mind in its object has been achieved.

6

It is maintained that the study and practice of Yoga purifies the body, improves the health, and strengthens the mind ; that, above all, it intensifies spiritual growth. Every person with sound mind and body is capable of attaining Yoga in some measure. The earlier in life the training is begun the better, but it is never too late to start its practices.

Since almost all men have their vulnerable points, it behoves the student to free his mind from malice, hatred, and all uncharitableness. He must restrain in himself all thought of evil, and avoid speaking of it. Any thought, regardless of its nature, can die from simple neglect. He must learn to be content, to accept joy without elation and sorrow without depression. When the mind wanders in search of pleasures of the senses, it must be brought back by the conviction that of all joys that of meditation is the greatest. He must ever be aware that the mind is an internal organ of sensation, and that it cannot maintain itself in the stream of life against the tide. It must work with it, but not be a part of it or be carried away by it.

Every effort must be used to purify and strengthen the mind. Sheer persistence will eliminate error in the long run. Ignorance is destroyed by the unbroken practice of discrimination; earnestness is the best gift of mental power. By constant introspection and by following the highest instincts, man can save himself from the bondage of this existence.

Regardless of the course a man's life may take, his very existence is the product of dynamic thought. It is the guiding force of all that he is or can hope to be. It is the beginning and the end of his suffering. It is the power that binds, and the power that frees him. If he is fond of a woman, it is the spirit of salaciousness that confuses him. If he is angry, it is the spirit of rage that seduces him. If he is covetous, it is the spirit of greed that deludes him. But, in the final analysis, it is the mind that acts as his enemy and not the spirit of the things. The secret of true happiness consists in considering all objects a source of grief. Ignorant people grow more ignorant all the while because they choose to dwell within their ignorance. Let the wise man shun the pain that has not yet come. This will hold him prepared for present joy and future suffering.

The Meaning of Yoga

Thoughts, good or bad, are like seeds. They will grow in soil that is fertile. One should meditate on wisdom in order to produce goodness not previously existing. The goodness that already exists can be increased if the attention of the mind is fixed on it, to the exclusion of evil.

The measure of such discipline is the measure of success or failure. The great need is mastery over self. By it one will grow content, without it one will deteriorate. With a disciplined mind, the touch is sure, the step firm, the vision sharp, the memory precise, the word positive, the thought clear, and silence itself wisdom. The disciplined body is unconscious of itself, and is the perfect servant.

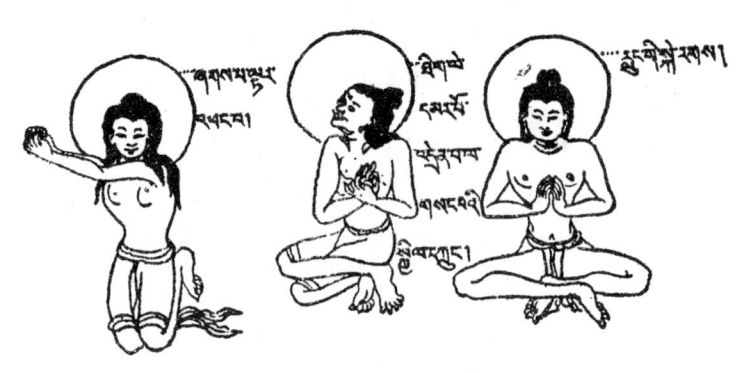

CHAPTER VI

SOME RULES FOR THE YOGIC DISCIPLE

I

QUITE often, even those who have faith in Yoga look upon it as something mysterious, something dangerous, something beyond their hope of attaining. This is especially true when one merely entertains the idea of a want or a future desire and never puts forth the effort to attain it. A great deal can be accomplished by earnest effort, and it is the purpose of this volume to offer the knowledge and the methods by which the prospective student may advance on the road to becoming a Yogi.

In the East the Yogi will devote the whole of his time to practice in order that he can by intensive training arrive rapidly at a measure of perfection. His mind is entirely given up to Yoga. It is clear that, considering conditions in the West, the Occidental must proceed more slowly, stretching his training over a greater period of time. When he has reached a degree of mastery, he can proceed with something of the enthusiasm of the Oriental. Time and perseverance are definitely necessary to demonstrate the value of Yoga. It has already been made evident that morality, practice, and discipline are the essential prerequisites of all Yoga.

In order to purify his soul, the Yogi courts silence, tranquillity, repose, solitude, moderation in eating and drinking. His ten rules of conduct are: Non-injury, truth, non-stealing, continence, forgiveness, endurance, compassion, meekness, sparse diet, and silence. As control over self is gained, faith becomes firmly established.

By persistent right living and adaptability one makes himself ready to permit the current of life to pass through him. Only practice and work will provide benefits, which no teacher can impart any more than he can impart the power of reason. The teacher can only point the way. As ripened fruit is always preceded by the budding and flowering, so is self-unfoldment of the Yogi preceded by self-development. As one's training deepens, the landmarks of worldliness become more and more faint, and a new creation with new scenes, new language, new thoughts, new aspirations and delights dawns upon the inward eye of the devotee.

From the very beginning the student must have faith in his understanding and faith in himself. By faith is meant that condition of mind which believes that it can and will accomplish the seemingly impossible. At the same time he must never lose the sense that man is in the dark, and that everything he thinks, says and does is nothing more nor less than a groping in this darkness towards some remote and as yet invisible light. Success and liberation are the goal. The method pursued is realistic enough; there is nothing supernatural or magical about it. It is labour, and again labour. Steady practice with regularity. Spasmodic spurts of intense activity will lead nowhere, whether in Yoga or in other endeavours. This must be remembered: if the student is too soon disappointed because he sees no visible results to which he has been impatiently looking forward, and, consequently, arrives at the conclusion that there is nothing in Yoga, the fault is all his own, not Yoga's.

2

It is next to impossible in the West to obtain guidance from someone who is competently trained in the art of Yoga. It was the realization of this urgent need that had brought me to India. To be sure, no little literature on

Yoga is available, and it is not to be denied that if one has an intense desire it is possible to learn some of the simpler rudiments of this esoteric art. It is equally certain, however, that Yogic practices of a higher order cannot be accomplished except under the guidance of an expert in such practices. The highly technical nature of these practices calls for verbal explanation and visual demonstration from a qualified Guru.

I have already indicated that the deserving disciple is hardly less rare than the qualified mentor. My Tantrik friend made it quite clear that the mere fact that I had given up a chosen career for which I had been trained and had come all the way to India to dedicate my life to learning the teachings of Yoga was not in itself sufficient to qualify me for becoming a Yogic disciple. Again and again he put me to the test. At every turn I was discouraged. It was impressed upon me that it was far better that I never begin than fail in my attempt. He was anxious to assure himself that mine was not a blind enthusiasm.

"How long will it take to acquire success in the practice of Yoga?" was the question I did not fail to put to my Tantrik mentor. And I received the answer that there could be no hard-and-fast rule applicable to all, since men's capacities were different. Indeed, it is one of the tasks of Yoga to indicate how these varying capacities can best be fostered to develop all the useful, natural powers in man. Man rarely makes the most of the stock he has won from the past. But he has great quantities of dormant energy, which Yoga helps to transmute into active, functional energy, so that man may become an independent, self-reliant, efficient being. When one's course has been determined and rightly directed, there will slowly and certainly take place in his body a molecular change. In the course of six months this change will achieve a corresponding change in his habits. And, of course, there will be a definite expansion in the powers of his mind. As the force within him becomes awakened, his state of consciousness will

Some Rules for the Yogic Disciple

change, and he will cease to be lonely, his fears will vanish, and happiness will be within his grasp.

The inherent endowment bestowed by life cannot be increased immediately for one's use. This can happen only after a long and arduous training, carefully and intelligently prepared. The means and the end are to be considered, so that method and goal may be perfectly balanced. The molecular perfection of man, advocated by Yoga, may be attained only after a prolonged period of exertion. And at the very beginning the disciple must qualify himself by ridding his body and his mind of such hindrances as I have already indicated.

To practise Yoga one must give up the eating of sour, sharp, and salty things, one must give up stimulating foods and foods tending to constipation; one must eschew gluttony, fasting, and starvation. One must avoid day sleeping or dozing, long journeys, all manner of bodily exertion; also bathing in an atmosphere that is chilling and sitting before the fire. One must keep away from the society of the evil-minded, the companionship of women; one must not make any distinction between relatives and outsiders. One must eliminate hatred, envy, pride, excitement, quarrelling, cruelty, falsehood, deceit, garrulousness, unpleasant speech, hostility towards any person or any thing, giving discomfort or pain to the body.

On the positive side, the disciple must wear comfortable clothing, keep his body internally and externally clean. He should be an early riser, cultivating regular habits. He should be careful of his health. The purity of the body is essential. He should be fearless, charitable, forgiving, steady, prayerful, anxious to do good to others and to pay homage to his instructors.

Power—I cannot stress this too often—develops like any other faculty, by the exercise of it. The "shalts" and "shalt-nots" of Yoga must be obeyed, and both one and the other are matters of restraint, and restraint itself implies a degree of courage. I was told to measure myself by the standard of my restraint. Those that most often fail in life are men and women who will not obey themselves. They cannot hold to a chosen course of action. They lose their grip. They fail their own hearts, the promise they have made themselves. But a standard may be raised if the person will but devote even a small fraction of his time to concentrated reflection on the nature of the True Self.

Aspirants to Yoga may be said to be of four kinds: mild, moderate, ardent, and super-ardent.

For the mild, Mantra Yoga is prescribed. For the moderate—Laya Yoga. For the ardent—Hatha Yoga. But the super-ardent is entitled to all forms of Yoga.

If the moderate disciple is steady-minded, independent, and energetic, he may attain his rewards in eight years or more. If the ardent disciple is the sort of man who is free from defects of blind emotions, not easily confused, and keeps his endeavours secret, he may, with steady persistence, receive his reward in six years or more. The super-ardent disciple may complete his practices in three years or more. These periods refer to final perfection of the art within Jiva's (soul's) limits.

3

I was very much confused when my Tantrik mentor began talking about different kinds of Yoga. I asked him to define for me, once and for all, the varieties of Yoga; for the books I had read on the subject were anything but illuminating.

He went on to explain that all of them were seeking the same goal, and more or less in the same way, just as in my own country all schools had the object of educating the student, yet employed a variety of systems and methods. He observed that some of them were called progressive schools. He pointed out that each had been planned to meet the requirements of a certain type of student. The same held true in the field of physical training in our country. The common purpose of all methods is to develop the individual physically, yet we know that one system requires the student to

Some Rules for the Yogic Disciple

work with heavy weights, while another—on the ground that this method is too strenuous for some persons—offers the student a set of setting-up exercises, designed to develop a measure of strength in him before he undertakes the practice of the more vigorous system. The same holds true of Yoga, whose various systems have been organized to meet the different capacities of the different students. This is one reason why the Guru must devote so much time to studying the potentialities of the pupil before proceeding to put him to work.

As I have already said, the four main forms of Yoga (according to the accepted Text) are Mantra Yoga, Hatha Yoga, Laya Yoga, and Raja Yoga. Other names, such as Bhakti Yoga, Karma Yoga, Jnana Yoga, Yantra Yoga, Dhyana Yoga, Shakti Yoga, Kundalini Yoga, and Samadhi Yoga, are not actually separate and distinct types of Yoga, but rather have reference to special actions or forms of disciplines within these four types.

There is a broader meaning to Yoga than is commonly supposed. Indeed, it will be found that most persons are practising Yoga in one form or another at all times; strictly speaking, Yoga is nothing more nor less than the rules of life. Such rules, however, are practised without system, without real direction, and it is the function of Yoga to provide this system, so that life may be conducted in the light of method instead of in the shadow of confusion. People who go to worship regularly in the churches are practising Bhakti Yoga, those who derive spiritual nourishment from music are practising Mantra Yoga, those who seek joy and solace in mental activities are following the path of Jnana Yoga, and those who train the body for their happiness are in a mild way practising Hatha Yoga.

I can go on interminably pointing out how Yoga exists everywhere. Yet it is a fact that Yogis are scarce, if not actually non-existent. What is wrong with the West is that there is no spiritual integration between a man's every-day life and his ultimate goal. Everything is at loose ends. He has his religion on Sundays, his mental training each morning, his physical training from four o'clock to sundown, and then he tries to be happy the rest of the day the best he can. The East teaches us that we must have our religion twenty-four hours a day for three hundred and sixty-five days a year, throughout our entire life. This does not mean that we are to follow empty forms of worship. The worship of the twentieth century is centred in action, but it should be action guided by the intelligence toward the common goal of all humanity. Everyone should awaken that creative flow of consciousness and bathe in it until the end. The Yogi abhors the thought of leaving it even for the few hours of sleep each day.

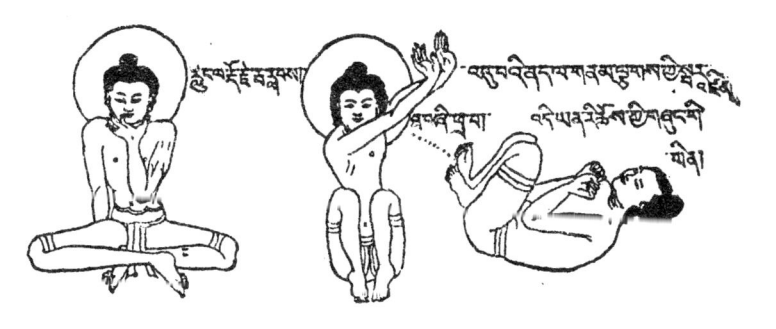

CHAPTER VII

"MORE IN HEAVEN AND EARTH . . ."

I

IN order to aid the student, it might be helpful to speak briefly of the four main forms of Yoga.

Mantra Yoga is a system concerned with the use of sound. The word "Mantra," from the Sanskrit, is a combination of the root "Man," to think, and of "Tra," liberation. Mantra has two sub-divisions: Kriya (action) and Bhava (feelings). Its spiritual function is to confer happiness in this world and eternal bliss in Liberation. On the ritualistic side, worship and devotion are predominant. The more esoteric side of Mantra Yoga can be taught only by a qualified teacher. No other can provide one with workable mantras, as the art is very technical, and there are but few Gurus who possess such training. Intellective processes are here supplemented by such auxiliaries as Hatha Yoga.

The word "Hatha" is combined from the syllables "Ha," the Sun, and "Tha," the Moon. These are symbolic of the personal and the universal consciousness. The combination of the two signifies Yoga.

Hatha affirms that concentration and Samadhi can be attained by the purification of the human body and by certain exercises. In this form of Yoga, stress is laid on breathing exercises, known as Pranayama. The first process in Hatha Yoga is to seek the perfection of the physical body, to make it a fitting instrument in which the mind can function. The relation between the physical shell of the body and the mind belongs, or should belong, to the subtle harmonies of life ; the interaction of the two is so curious, so involved in solemn mystery, that it is not strange that the specialists in Hatha Yoga should have conceived the idea that certain specific physical training would induce the desired mental transformation. It is erroneous to look upon Hatha Yoga as mere physical training having no spiritual counterpart ; yet some of its critics go so far as to assert that Hatha Yoga runs counter to the higher forms of Yoga. This perverse notion is due to the failure to see the relationship between Hatha Yoga and the higher discipline of Yoga. It is impossible to follow any form of Yoga until the student has gained a thorough understanding of the Yamas and Niyamas, which are the first steps in Hatha Yoga. A Hatha Yogi cares for his body simply because it is the only instrument he has to help him reach his spiritual goal ; therefore, it is a prerequisite to Raja Yoga.

The third form of Yoga, known as Laya Yoga—" Laya " means absorption—consists of fixing the attention upon certain subtle sounds in the body, until the mind becomes absorbed in them. These sounds manifest themselves during certain breathing exercises, and are known as Pranic sounds. Laya Yoga is the forgetting of the objects of the senses ; it functions to prevent sense desires from coming into existence again ; it also operates to crush all thought activity. Its achievement is the highest form of contemplation, and is infinitely precious, for it makes possible the direct perception of Self.

The transcendent form of Yoga, however, is Raja Yoga, so called because it is founded upon the eight steps which lead to Samadhi ; it is purely mental discipline. It actually utilizes all forms of Yoga, and is generally considered to be the ultimate form of all Yoga.

2

My host proceeded to supply me with a more clear understanding of the basic principles of the require-

"*More in Heaven and Earth . . .*"

ments of Hatha Yoga than I yet possessed. There are seven steps in the practice of Hatha Yoga:

1. The body is first purified.
2. The body is then made strong and enduring. This method has been called the science for the training of hardiness and vital powers.
3. The body is then made to remain still, motionless.
4. Patience is established, for the sake of faith and confidence.
5. The body is made light.
6. The body uses its powers objectively.
7. The body uses its powers subjectively, so that the mind may become unattached.

Purification provides the proper standard of health. Asana makes the body strong and durable. Mudra keeps it still. Pranayama makes it light. Pratyahara gives it patience. Dharana gives control over the senses objectively. Dhyana provides the subjective control.

Genuine devotees of Yoga see as its aim the union between the Jiva (individual or embodied consciousness) and the Paramatma (universal or transcendental consciousness). Hatha Yoga is referred to as the "Supporting Tortoise," and one is cautioned to practise this Yoga system very privately. One is permitted to reveal it only to those who have faith in the system and seek after introspection. After the treasure has been attained, it may be taught to another; but until then secrecy is ordained. Hatha Yoga is supposed to be the shortest method for the purification and control of the body.

One of the first functions of Hatha Yoga is to resolve the doubts of the mind. It calls upon the disciple to observe an act of the Will, the ability to say Yes or No. Then it enjoins unity upon the body and the mind, in order that they can co-operate in a very complete sense. If the body grumbles, the mind soothes it and makes it obey; if the mind grumbles, the body pleads with it, prevailing upon it to go on.

These are initial steps, without which further steps

are out of the question. Once accomplished, they indicate that the body has been thoroughly purified, and has become one with the desire of the mind to practise Yoga; in short, it has become fit for Yoga. The next stage is concerned with knowledge of Self, both mental and physical. It consists of an analysis of every desire, which must be traced to its source. It aims at a thorough study of one's temperament and tendencies. It is necessary to follow with precision the state of bodily health, and to have knowledge of proper food and medicine for the maintenance of this standard. After this, measures must be taken to prevent oneself from becoming entangled with the Ego; it is unfitting that the disciple should become attached to the phenomena of his creation, or that he should exhibit pride in his achievement. The final stage is that unconscious state which the Yogi can induce at will and in which he can remain indefinitely. These last steps, whose functions I have explained in this paragraph, may be attained after mastering the six practical systems of Asana, Pranayama, Pratyahara, Dharana, Dhyana, and Samadhi.

3

Nerve culture is the primary aim of Hatha practices. It is certain that nerves are the most important fibres of our body. Lack of endurance may be ascribed to the unhealthy condition of the nerves. Mental balance, too, reflects a good motor and muscular balance. Stable nerves provide calm and efficiency. It is the function of Hatha Yoga exercises to improve the degenerated nerve supply and to restore a diseased organ to health.

The importance of this can scarcely be exaggerated when it is realized that degenerative diseases of the heart, kidneys, arteries, and nervous system are to-day on the increase. It is said that two million persons die yearly in the United States. Three million are always ailing in bed, and forty thousand die annually of stomach cancer. In a period when a race shows indications of physical degeneration, vice and luxury show greater prevalence, and there is a demand for artificial stimulation. All exhausted natures will testify to this. In a sense, it may be said that thousands and tens of thousands of persons who are presumed to have died natural deaths have really committed a sort of progressive suicide.

To acquire a perfect working circulation of the blood and to master the appetites may seem to be a very lowly beginning for a great quest. Yet it cannot be too emphatically stressed that this work, having a spiritual purpose, is not to be confused with any system of physical culture, with bodily accomplishment as the primary goal. Many of the Yoga practices may seem puerile and useless, and even ridiculous. Nevertheless, they are an essential part of the system and all calculated for spiritual unfoldment. There should be no scorn for little things, which are, after all, symptomatic of the whole ; and in a state of perfection they hold a place as important as the big things.

It may be laid down as a law that the body and mind are interdependent, and in a harmonious human being they sustain each other. And Yoga practices are, in effect, a realistic recognition of this law. On the physical side, the highest good of Yoga is to eliminate all disorders of the system, to produce the highest standard of health, and to direct nervous energy into any action desired. On the mental side, it is to control all the desires, and to guide them according to one's will. Its practices aim at the improvement of the nerves, glands, and muscles, which are responsible for the health of the different organs, and at the removal of offending matter, and the oxygenation of the blood. Disorders of metabolism are corrected in the main by the remarkable elimination derived from the practice of Pranayama. It is necessary to acquire perfect elimination before one can have the power to take in or assimilate. By elimination and the cleansing of the body, the divine element within one is increased, and one becomes a better being physically, mentally, and morally.

F

4

Practices on the physical body are essential only where impurities exist in the Nadis (channels through which nervous energy passes), and since no one is physically perfect, it is advisable not to neglect wholly such practices as are helpful, if only as a precautionary measure. There are two processes of purifying the Nadis. One is a mental process which includes breathing exercises; the other is a physical process. Some teachers, however, assert that Pranayama (breathing exercises) is all the therapeutics required to burn up the impurities of the body and that the Nadis will be purified if the practices are maintained for three months without interruption. This practically means that from the beginning one must have already perfected the art of Yoga.

Before it is possible to practise Pranayama, it is essential that the disciple first rid his body of all excess Kapha (phlegm), because this excludes the Prana (breath or nervous energy) from the veins and nerves. This phlegm causes a befogged brain, defective speech, impure blood, and, in general, inhibits all bodily function. Yogic success cannot be attained until the Nadis are cleansed of all obstructing matter. The nerves in their natural state are covered with impurities which must be removed before there can be any real accomplishment in Pranayama.

Among the three most important Nadis is Sushumna, which is centrally situated inside the spinal column, extending from the brain to the pelvic plexus. The lower part of Sushumna descends through the centre of the mass of nerves in the sacral and coccygeal section of the vertebræ. The upper part goes inside the cranium and extends to the region of the foramen Monroe known in Yoga literature as the " Door of Brahma." This great Nadi is the sustainer of the body, supporting all the Nadis, leading the Yogi to the path of mental abstraction and salvation. Inside this central Nadi the Yogi identifies an invisible Nadi known in the West as the fibre of Reissner, but which is known here as Chittra (the Heavenly Passage, in Sanskrit). It is by means of this fine threadlike nerve that Kundalini (energy) is said to move upward through the several nerve plexus of the spinal column.

The sympathetic nervous system has its main connection with Sushumna at the solar plexus. Ida and Pingala are two nerves outside of the spinal column thought to be the gangliated cords of the sympathetic system. These two Nadis join with Sushumna in the cranium at the position between the two eyebrows known as the Ajna Chakra (centre), Ida going to the left nostril and Pingala to the right. In their downward course along the spine these two Nadis cross each other several times, as well as communicate freely with the spinal nerve, terminating at the base of the spine in the pelvic plexus at a point horizontal to the hip bone. The regions within the spinal column, where the Nadis cross each other, are the Mystic Circles and are called Chakras.

5

I was learning much about the aims of Yoga, yet I must admit I was beginning to feel restless in the jungle shelter of my Tantrik host. I had come to India to practise Yoga, and not learn about Yoga. I had not the time to quell my Western temperament, and was impatient to come to grips with the problem I had come to solve, to discover the meaning that life was to have for me. If it lay for me in Yoga, I wanted to get down to the practices of Yoga. My host did not profess to be a Yogi, but only a scholar of the philosophy of Yoga. He had devoted his life to the study of Tantrik literature, and, having been initiated, he possessed a deep insight into its unfathomable mysteries. All Tantrik literature is written in such a highly symbolic form that only the initiate who possesses the Key, so to speak, is able to interpret it. My background, training, and interest were sufficient for him to talk freely to me about matters he felt were within my comprehension. He made it quite clear, however, that I should have to be initiated before it would be possible for me to understand the more esoteric aspects of the Yogic practices. He was not particularly cheerful about my prospects of finding a Guru capable of preparing me for initiation. These higher Tantrik teachings had apparently fallen into disuse even in India. Wars and the trying climate had caused a deterioration in the manuscripts, while the accelerated spread of Western ideas and attendant materialism had pushed the teachers out of India, so that at this time the only available teachers were reported to be in Tibet. Moreover, before the great Mogul invasion, an army of Tibetan scholars came to India and carried back to Tibet with them the great bulk of manuscripts containing the ancient teachings.

The idea of going to Tibet to make contacts with the Tantrik teachers attracted me immeasurably. The ancient teachers, preserved in the sixty-four volumes of the Tantra, books jealously guarded by the Lamas through the ages, seemed to hold an unaccountable lure for me, and I began to dream of going to Tibet and bringing back a set of these precious books. I asked my host why it was that some of those who had been initiated had not gone to Tibet and brought back the teachings to India. He explained that even the Indian was forbidden to enter the Forbidden Land; indeed, it was harder for a Bengali than for any other foreigner to get into Tibet. Moreover, nothing would be gained by going to Tibet unless one was first initiated as a Tantrik, as only a Tantrik was likely to get into contact with the true teachers. A barrier had been created by the circumstance that those who made the effort to enter Tibet had been persons interested in adventure rather than in the spiritual aspect of things. Still another difficulty had been that even persons qualified as Tantriks were for the most part individuals raised in low altitudes and in a hot climate; they lacked the hardihood to undertake so arduous a journey in the lofty and brisk Tibetan altitudes. Only a person who could meet all the requirements might undertake a journey with any measure of physical and spiritual success.

After a fortnight, my friend, having become assured of my sincerity and ability, said that he was ready to take me to a man who might become my Guru. No sooner said than done; we resolved promptly to return to my friend's home in the city.

6

I no longer felt a stranger on my return to Calcutta. Something of India had already entered my soul, and become an integral part of me. And on the very evening of our return we set out to visit my prospective Guru, who was known as the Swamaji. It was a journey of some hours up India's sacred river, the Ganges.

The Swamaji was less familiar with the English language than my Tantrik friend, who was proficient in it. I managed, however, to get along with him, until we touched upon the more abstract and technical subjects. Both men were versed in Sanskrit literature and, indeed, had contributed to it. Its content is so highly specialized that it is well-nigh impossible to translate it into another tongue. Our first visit was a brief one. After my Tantrik friend had supplied an appraisal of me, the result of our fortnight's association, the Swamaji consented to undertake my initiation. We then returned to the city after a very delightful ride down the quiet river in the full light of the moon.

After further meetings with the Swamaji, some time elapsed before I received word from him to the effect that a certain date and hour would be very auspicious for my initiation, and that he would be then at home to receive me. He had previously given me my preparatory instructions.

Not to be late, I started early up the river, and on arrival stopped for some time on its banks awaiting the hour when I might put in an appearance before the

Swamaji. The gentle stir of the slow current on a warm evening, and the passing gusts of a cool breeze, filled me with unaccountable awe ; my emotions ran high. All the yearnings I had ever experienced seemed on this evening to be dammed up in me, waiting for release in my first initiation, which was to be the gleaning of my first inner understanding. The purpose of this initiation was to awaken the creative flow within, to free the mind of prejudices, to make the soul receptive to all things in quest of Eternal Happiness.

It seemed so strange that I had come so far from the lonely deserts of Arizona to this devout land, from an environment so young to a culture so old. What had planted the seeds within me of this desire to come here? What had called me to this Land of Mystery? Why was I being accepted? It was clear, or so it seemed to me now, that all my effort to gain some understanding of the Laws of Life had not been in vain. The old saying that when the pupil was ready the teacher would appear flashed upon my mind, and I felt there was truth in it. I knew I was on the verge of being liberated, on the path to verify by experience what I had learned in theory. Already I was realizing how the emotions expand while the intellect contracts ; for I had almost become unaware of the passage of time. The initiation was to begin at midnight. It was to be the start of a new life for me, of spiritual rebirth. The shackles of the personal consciousness would be forever removed. I would directly perceive the universal manifestation of the Divine Law.

7

The hour for my appearance before the Swamaji had arrived. I was welcomed at the entrance of his abode by others who were to participate with me in the ceremony. I was handed two pieces of cloth, one a Dhoti (a cloth to cover the lower part of the body), the other a Chadar (a cloth to cover the upper part of the body). They were dyed a brick-red, and were not without symbolical significance. As soon as I had changed into this apparel, I was ushered into the presence of the Swamaji, who was in the company of five other Tantriks.

I must make it clear that, having taken the vow of secrecy, I am permitted to speak only of the formal aspects of the ceremony which is regarded as highly esoteric.

As the master of the Chakra (sacred circle), the Swamaji was supreme, and his wish had to be obeyed in every instance during the ceremony of initiation. He was seated on a slightly raised seat before the deity of the Chakra. The rest of us were seated in Asana (sacred posture) in a semicircle about him; I was on his left, the second from the end. The Chakra was scented with the many flowers gathered for this rite, as well as sprinkled with scented water. Everything there was for the purpose of enabling the Sadhaka (worshipper) to awaken his inner consciousness. First there was a period of silence, during which I was to make an offering of my ignorance in order that I might become receptive to what the Swamaji was going to pass on to me. This is the natural law in the world of teacher and disciple. For, surely, there can be no need for a Guru (spiritual teacher) unless one is ignorant. One may be well educated in many subjects, yet be in complete ignorance in the field of Sadhana (spiritual practices). The pupil has not the least notion, or even the suspicion of a notion, as to what the Guru will teach him. Spiritual knowledge is not to be tested by the same standards as worldly knowledge. After I had meditated for a short while, the purpose of the ceremony was explained to me. Having sprinkled me with consecrated ritual water, the Swamaji then gave us a Mantra to repeat, following which he recited chants to cast a spell over me, in order to awaken the universal consciousness within. Then he made known the manifestation of the universal consciousness in its infinite number of forms. He took one aspect at a time, and before each, Mantras were recited, in order to induce a wholly different feeling, soon dispelled by understanding brought about by a simple truth that he would utter and dwell upon for a short while.

Thus the hours flew by, as I was being born into a new world of knowledge. Finally, the Swamaji's head and my own were covered over with a cloth, as the Swamaji whispered seven times into my left ear and seven times into my right the Mantra that was to be kept inviolate in the recesses of my mind, never to cross my lips in utterance. As the cloth was removed and I felt the dawn of this rebirth, the heart slowly awakened to a silent joy. The darkness of doubt was forever dispelled. I was free.

On the termination of the Chakra, I rose and made the sacrificial offering within my means. Then we broke my fast with a light feast. It was necessary that a fast be kept from sundown the day before my initiation until after the ceremony. The Swamaji's attendant had prepared some very tasty food and brought it into the Chakra. It was he who had arranged the Chakra and the instruments of worship for my initiation.

The dawn was about to break, and as boats were no longer available for my return to the city, one of the Tantriks who lived in the country drove me over a rather long and circuitous route to a place where I could get a gharry to take me back to my abode. I arrived there just in time for Chota Hazri.

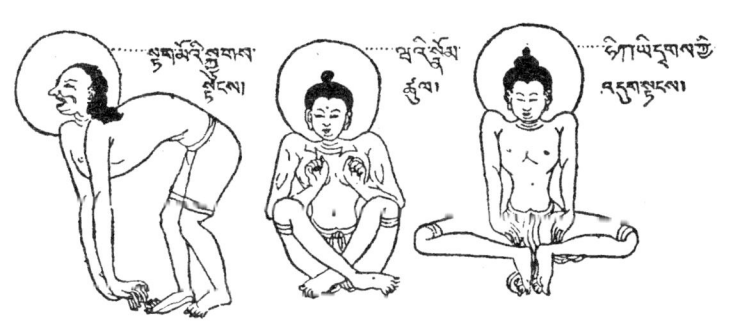

CHAPTER VIII

APPRENTICESHIP OF THE MIND

I

WHEN I went to the home of my Tantrik friend to tell him of my initiation, he received me with the welcoming arms of a father who meets his son after he has graduated from college.

The real work, however, was only about to begin. It was up to me to put my recent experience into practice. And it was pleasant to talk my plans over with one who, in spite of our brief acquaintance, seemed like a lifelong friend. The next step was one which required some deliberation. Success now wholly depended on my own capacity, on my ability to discern the Universal thread of consciousness in this welter of earthly existence. The Truth had been revealed to me, but I had yet to learn its function in our dynamic world of struggle and action. To retreat into the jungle again with my friend would not advance me an inch. It was necessary that I travel among men.

There is no place on earth where it is possible to find such a mixture of human beings as in India. It offers the greatest array of religious beliefs to be found in any one spot in the world. Every one of these beliefs is the outgrowth of a mind that has tried to interpret the Truth as he has seen it. This was a living laboratory. It was not for me to discover wherein each cult was wrong, but rather where they all led to the same goal. Through it all I was expected to perceive the eternal groping of Man in that blind effort which we call spiritual evolution. In other words, I was to tear away the veils of Maya (illusion) and uncover that Truth which is everywhere present. How was I to glean this understanding, was my question; how to know the Truth and reconcile it with the false?

And thus it came about that a plan was made for me to tour all India, and on the eve of starting on my journey my Tantrik friend and I went to say good-bye to my new Guru, the Swamaji. I had scarcely arrived at his house when I began to ply him with questions, all dealing with the problem of developing the mind according to their teachings and making it possible to comprehend all appearances in the light of my new knowledge. I was especially eager to learn the Yogic attitude to the wonders in the realms of the mind. I was possessed of an abundance of enthusiasm which, from their point of view, was a dubious possession unless intelligently directed; otherwise, it was no more than a gust of wind. It was an excellent thing, however, with which to open the heart, and an open heart made possible true perception, always a matter of feeling. I learned this much from my initiation, if nothing more. Thus, it was now necessary for me to acquire a method by which I could always awaken the heart to listen to all that I wanted to know forever. One of the most efficacious ways was to direct the fires of enthusiasm into the heart.

2

In response to my questions, my Guru began his exposition on the mind, as it is understood by the Yogi. In any system of Yoga there is no differentiation between mind and matter, mind being merely the product of highly organized matter partaking of the qualities of both Spirit and Matter. All this mobile and immobile world is Mind, and when it attains Brahma (Supreme Consciousness) it ceases to work. Mind appears only in the living things that have breath (Prana). In man the Spirit (Atma) is most manifest. Being equipped with

Apprenticeship of the Mind

knowledge, he speaks what he knows, and he is conscious of what occurred yesterday and to-day. He is also conscious of the visible and the invisible. But in animals hunger and thirst are the principal knowledge.

The purpose of the mind is to ascertain. It is a sort of reflecting surface, the bridge between the lower and the higher Self—Intellect below, Intelligence above. It is the directing power behind everything. It is the mind that commits sin, demeritorious acts; at the same time sin can never touch it if it knows how to retain its proper function. When dominated by sensuous desires and images, it cannot reflect or reveal its innermost faculty, that of Spirit. Power is its greatest asset, and its cultivation by proper methods will result in a force, a capacity, and an elevation which have not yet been realized by Western savants.

In the ordinary individual the mind is an entirely uncontrolled function. The average human being is a slave to his thoughts. He has no power over his thought life, he cannot drive away those thoughts which are undesirable and he cannot command those he desires. For this reason the disciple with sensual appetites is excluded. Only purity of mind induces concentration and meditation.

Mind is master of the senses, and breath is master of mind. As the bee follows the queen, so does the mind follow Prana. External forces affect Prana directly, the mind can be affected indirectly through Prana. The mind can never be restrained without restraining the breath; mental activity keeps pace with the respiration. As the waves roll on and on when driven by the wind and cease rolling when the wind grows still, so does the mind grow quiescent when the breath is controlled. As long as breath is restrained within the body, the mind is undisturbed. Hence, if the mind is to be steady and peace enjoyed, the breath must be regulated. When the respiration is agitated, it affects the heart, and this in turn agitates the mind, whose perceptions thus become clouded and stupefied.

Breathing is lessened in proportion as the mind is absorbed. This means they are equal in their activities, one beginning where the other begins. Hence, by the control of the breath, the mind and death are conquered. When the modifications of the thinking principle become suspended, one is then a Yogi, a possessor of pure knowledge.

To work properly, the brain should have a normal pulse. Blood pressure and its rhythm are the criteria by which this is to be judged, since the pumping of the heart determines the rate of active thought. Normally we should have four pulse beats to each inhalation, and four to each exhalation; this is rhythmic breath. Rhythmic breathing simply means the maintenance of this scale of proportion between the pulse and the breath. On the other hand, we do not inhale the same quantity of air that we exhale, the proportion being regulated by the demands of the body, which is never the same. The pulse should be thirty-two per minute when one is inhaling eight times a minute. If the pulse exceeds this, then we know that the physical man rules. But if the breath is greater, then the mental man predominates. All is timed at the rate of one to four. Rhythmic breathing means the control of the time value of things, putting an end to our emotions in relation to time. This indicates control over the emotions, making it possible to gauge a particular emotion to a particular time.

In Yoga the subject of the mind resolves itself into three parts: (1) Mind; (2) Its modifications; (3) The mode of restraining it. All questions on the mind finally and naturally fall into the third division. There are two means of control which Yoga teaches: (1) Specific practices; (2) Freedom from desires.

3

Generally the mind keeps running restlessly from object to object in the length and breadth of space, revealing that it is of a superficial character. How then is it to be made to go to the depth of space? If it is to plunge deep into space, it must first be made one-pointed. For illustration, we may consider the following example: While one is swimming about on the surface of the water, how is he to plunge deep into its depths? First, he must cease swimming back and forth. Then, stationing himself at one point on the water's surface, he suspends his breath and dives in. Similarly, the mind should cease its wanderings on the surface of the superficies of space and engage itself in concentrating upon one point or object, then dive in. Then only will it be able to "think deeply." The ordinary man can only guess or infer, he learns by trial and friction; but the Yogi cognizes directly. It is the primary object of Yoga to make the mind one-pointed, to render it capable of holding a habitual attitude of attention on any object it will. Without form or shape, it yet assumes the form of the thing it thinks. It is a sort of natural substance, receptive to whatever object comes to it by way of the senses, and reflecting all things as in a mirror. The mind makes a tactile contact, as do the senses, creating its own reality. Conditioned by the contact, feelings arise. What one feels, one perceives; what one perceives, one thinks about. And what one thinks about, one may become obsessed with.

Every mental state has a corresponding respiration. As an illustration, consider the mental act of listening to catch a faint and indistinct sound; breathing is suspended. It is impossible to listen while breathing deep and full. In melancholy, the respiration is suspended; in surprise, man catches his breath spasmodically. Every action of concentration means so much suspension. When one wants to lift a heavy weight, the first thing done is the suspension of breath. Tell a lad he cannot lift a rock that lies before him, and, if he accepts the challenge, he instinctively assumes an erect attitude, and, then taking a full breath, he triumphantly raises the rock. There is a practical and profound philosophy in what he does. He first forms the idea of strength in his mind, then he translates it into a bodily attitude, and finally into its form of respiration; ultimately there is a vigorous muscular contract, and the rock is lifted. Breath determines the pressure behind all emotions, activities, and circulation; it has to do with feelings, life, senses. Its influence is far greater than we ever suspect.

In profound thought the respiration is slow and deep; in intense thought the mind stops the flow of Prana (breath). And it may be observed that one's respiration has, for a time, been stopped, or greatly suspended, when all of a sudden one finds a need for more air and takes one or more deep breaths until the need has been satisfied, after which the mind may again become fixed. The scientist, when he is lost in concentration, is actually practising Pranayama, but his Kumbhaka (suspension) is usually external. Thus we find that all our moods, thoughts, and feelings are constantly regulating the body respiration. Observation of this led the ancients to believe that if one could control his breath, one could control one's mind.

There are two causes of the activity of the mind. One is desire, the other Prana (breath). The destruction of one means the destruction of the other. Yet it is well to remember that even when the mind is brought to a temporary standstill through the stopping of Prana, the mind will still continue to dwell on its favourite desires. Hence, for its complete control two things are required: indifference to desires and indifference to one's practice. Even when our desires are brought under control, Prana agitates the mind and keeps it in constant motion. It is, therefore, necessary to bring both under control. If the mind is under control, the Chitta (feeling consciousness) is also under control, and there is no obstruction to the Intelligence that tries to flow through us.

4

The Self consists of Speech, Mind, and Breath. Since these are interdependent, by controlling the mind the breath and speech are controlled; or, if the breath is

Apprenticeship of the Mind

controlled, the mind and speech are brought under control. Day after day the mind awakens to Intelligence, and becomes completely capable of drawing on the Truth from the fountainhead that is within. Thus is Self almost wholly forgotten, and the human being who practises this wisdom feels for others as he would for himself. The purer the mind, the more sensitive it is to the slightest and remotest tendency of Prana toward change. In consequence, the Yogi is ever conscious of any impending change.

When the mind is brought to a single point, it is easy for it to go higher or deeper into the subject, or object, at hand. Everything must come to a point to achieve manifestation. For ordinary mortals, however, to suspend thought and merge the Self with the Spirit is as impossible as it is to stop the motion of the planets. Those Yogic practices which give the ability to identify oneself with any object and gain full knowledge of the thing or subject taken together are known as Samyama.

Training of the mind enables one to use his preconscious thoughts. By the ability to control the mind, occult powers may be acquired. The exercises of inner insight require tranquillity of mind; the individual never knows his true worth until his mind is slowed down or stopped entirely. This will permit the finer thoughts to rush in from the intuitive side. There should never be any strain in the operation of the mind. It should be an almost automatic performance. Violent effort is the mark of an inefficient mind. The individual mind blunders, while the Universal Mind works as competently as a finished writer, or expert musician, paying less and less attention to what he is doing, oblivious of the process, accomplishing without effort.

The Yogi adopts a special method to accelerate his evolution in the control of his mind, resorting to practices which will assist him in withdrawing his thoughts from all disturbing impressions in order that he can fix them upon a single object. Once he has attained perfect control over his mind, powers almost superhuman are his. Mind disappears on removing the knowable, and upon its disappearance only Atma, the Spirit, remains. The act of separating the mind from the body and uniting it with the Universal Mind is known as Mukti. There are three ways in which the mind can be brought under control: (1) Through itself; (2) Through Prana; (3) Through the organs of sense and action. The first process is called Dharma, which is right action, or that action which redeems the individual from the weakening tendencies of his age. It is the art of tuning the mind to special thoughts, the binding of the Chitta (the mind) to one place; thus is it purified by habituation. The second is by regulating the breath to which the mind is tied. The third method is by means of the discipline of the senses and action. The body being made motionless for three hours, the mind will follow suit. Body and mind are partners; control of the body gives also control of the mind.

Concentration upon a single thought has become to most of us as impossible as to apprehend a single musical note without harmonics. The helter-skelter life we are leading, with the multiplicity of things and interests breaking in upon us, makes it impossible to arrive at that intensity of thought which the Hindus call contemplation, and the attainment of which is the indispensable condition of all philosophical and religious speculation. Only now did I begin to grasp the purpose behind the instructions given me by my first Guru in America when I began my practices.

The mind must be trained to concentrate its attention upon the occupation of the moment. All ideas and memories having an interrelation should be brought together. The degree of stability of the impression is dependent upon the quantity of strength and duration put in the practice; half-hearted effort is never as beneficial as when the person is absorbed, even to the point of forgetfulness. The person who is too easy on himself will not get very far. The mind is slow to receive, but it is tenacious in retaining any impression sufficiently made.

5

The intellect is to the mind what the senses are to the body: a bureau of information in which facts are collected. It must not be confused with intelligence, though it be included in it. Intellect is used to obtain knowledge. It can do three things: Think, Remember, Imagine. Thinking takes place in the present; memory brings the past up to the present; imagination carries one into the future. Intellect is a function of the mind; intelligence is a thing above, and apart from, the mind. It is not a part of it. The mind is only an instrument through which the intelligence can be expressed. It is that which illumines, which gives comprehension.

The following five classifications of the mind, of very ancient origin, reminded me of a certain statement, "This earth is the insane asylum for all the other planets":

1. The insane state, wherein the mind is never calm, being constantly tossed on the sea of worldliness.

2. The mind always clouded by such dominant passions as anger, lust, vanity, covetousness, etc.

3. A state very much like the second, except for occasional lucid intervals. The first may be compared to a continued state of fever, the third to a remittent fever.

4. In this state the mind is steadily centred on one worthy object, avoiding the losing of itself in the whirl of this gross world.

5. A state in which the mind has no external or internal wants, but is supremely happy: a potential, immovable state.

It is the object of Yoga to calm the mind in the first stage, to banish worldliness from the second and third, with a view to the attainment of the fourth and fifth stages.

If a man discovers his mistakes and tries carefully to

correct them, the mistakes of themselves will cease to exist. Ignorance is destroyed only by the unbroken practice of discrimination: hence, earnestness is the best gift of mental power. Two things are essential in bringing about the control of the mind: control of Prana, and association. By association is meant disassociation with the longing for things and objects. In short, what is needed is the absence of attachment, complete indifference.

My Guru (the Swamaji) pointed out that, thanks to scientific research in my country, it has been satisfactorily demonstrated that the brain is nothing but an apparatus for burning sugar, which is transformed into electric currents, the nervous system distributing them throughout the body. The brain is merely a physiological mechanism which exists for the purpose of doing a particular piece of work. This mechanism has to be kept in proper order; it requires, indeed, more care than an ordinary machine, and receives less. If a person is to be rewarded in possessing it, he must see to it that it is constantly bathed in rich red blood ; only then will it maintain its highest standard of functioning.

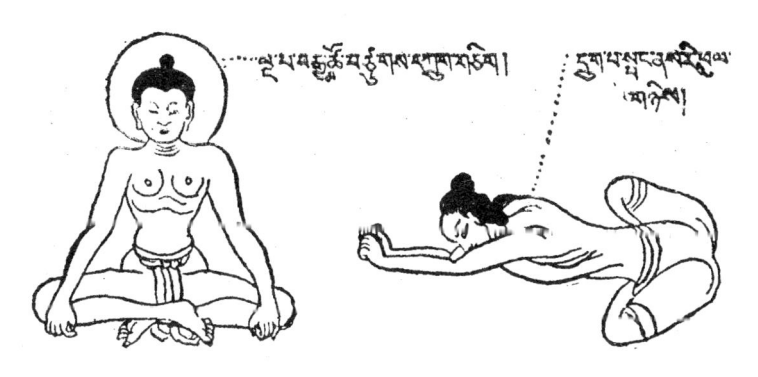

CHAPTER IX

CONSCIOUSNESS

I

THE idea of consciousness is of the utmost importance in the Yogic doctrine.

Most persons consider consciousness, mind, and intellect as equivalent. By consciousness they mean the sum total of all our impressions received through the physical side of our existence; hence, consciousness is not the highest form of experience. This consciousness—sense consciousness—begins with the first breath of life. It is co-eval and co-existent with our respiration throughout the entire cycle of our earthly existence, and will cease to exist with it. This consciousness is conditioned by the arising of differentiations as we grow. On the other hand, the impressions which we do not get through the physical side of existence are intuitive or instinctive. The instinctive side knows all about the conscious side, but the conscious side does not know anything about the instinctive side.

When one is awake, one knows that he has a body; he is aware of its parts and organs. But when one is asleep, the work of the body goes on without any conscious awareness of it. Hence, the first period of consciousness is the waking period, when all the senses are at their fullest activity. The second period is the dream state, the third the deep sleep, the fourth unconsciousness—or what might more properly be called the superconscious state. When impressions are repeated, and repeated through the senses, a sufficient number of times and over a sufficiently long period, they become instinctive. The highest character results from perfect co-ordination between the conscious and instinctive minds. Of these two functions of the mind, the thinking and the perceptive, the thinking can be stopped with relative ease, but the perceptive function it is extremely difficult to check.

Consciousness (as feeling) resides in the heart. It is analogous to a blackboard upon which things are written, or a film upon which the objective side is imprinted, an impression or thought moment (Writti, smallest unit of consciousness) upon the Chitta (feeling consciousness); it is the substratum on which all the faculties exist. When referring to the seat of trial, tribulation, pain, joy, happiness, and unhappiness, one automatically speaks of the heart, never the brain, which is the organ of the mind. One always says, "take it to heart," "peace of heart," "appealing to the heart," "heart of the doctrine," "learn by heart." On approach of sleep, the mind enters the coronary artery (Nadi of the heart), then the pericardium, then into the interior of the heart, which is its seat. The Cardiac plexus associated with the heart has a Chakra (centre) of eight petals; here is said to be the seat of the forces of the mind or Chitta. Feeling consciousness, and not logic, is the basis of human nature, the motive power behind human action. When thinking consciousness becomes suspended, feeling consciousness increases. Life itself is but consciousness lightly veiled. What is wanted is not consciousness under the limitation of the mind, but consciousness *per se*, consciousness free of hampering factors.

2

How is the mind to be cultivated? To cultivate anything, be it a plant, animal, or mind, is to make it grow and expand. Self-Culture is man's need, if he is to become a well-proportioned, vigorous, happy, harmonious being. Its practice has four stages: Physical, Mental, Moral, Spiritual. Each stage prepares the ground for improvement in the following stage.

To arrive at Self Mastery is a long, arduous effort, painful at the beginning but sweet at the end, like poison at the start but ending in ambrosia. Its rewards are serenity and happiness, from which knowledge is born. Thus is discipline shown to be a means to an end, and the end is Self-Control, which is the path to the highest manifestation in man. It is mental discipline that enables the great men of the world to rise into eminence. But it also counts in such matters as business. It is certain that success lies this way. The discipline should embrace the whole nature of man, his knowing, his desiring, and his willing. Yoga does this for one.

Better to illustrate the truth of what the Swamaji had been telling me and the substance of which I have just given, let me quote what Mr. J. Gallhuber has written concerning the selection of the men who were to take part in the British Mt. Everest Expedition:

> Will-power is the motor of great deeds. It is the secret of success of great men.
>
> It is the will-power that leads the scientist, the merchant, the artist, the sportsman, and also the mountain climber, out of the grey " common run " to great achievements.
>
> When the members of the British Mt. Everest Expedition were chosen, the task was faced of securing the participation of people with great energy.
>
> Hence an experiment was devised that made it possible to measure the will-power with some accuracy. This experiment, however, is a very serious matter and may be undertaken only after consultation with an expert physician and upon his advice.
>
> The procedure was as follows: The examination candidate was seated in a comfortable arm-chair with his clothes loosened. Then he drew a deep breath and was told to refrain absolutely from further breathing; that is, as long as he possibly could. However, he was permitted to exhale.
>
> The following phenomena became apparent: After 30 to

55 seconds a slight discomfort and the desire to breathe set in. This was followed by a period of more or less acute pain which increased in an extraordinarily quick manner and lasted about 40 to 80 seconds. Then an unusual exertion of self-control was necessary to suppress the breathing.

Then the pain gradually subsided, grew duller, and was easier to bear. At the same time the strain required to refrain from inhaling increased to an enormous degree, and after 3 to $5\frac{1}{2}$ minutes the person experimented upon fainted, if he had not already collapsed.

The length of time that man may hold out without inhaling furnishes a will-power scale that is well qualified for the purpose of comparison.

Therefore, if he is capable of eliminating inhalation until he faints, he possesses the greatest possible will-power, and seems eminently qualified for record performances.

3

It should be thought very strange if one's hands and feet refused to behave, or behaved in a manner which showed that their owner had no control over them. Yet that is how too often human beings allow their most delicate instrument, the mind, to behave. It is truly a deplorable and absurd state of affairs, and it is the endeavour of Yoga to set it right, by means of Self Discipline.

Much has already been said about the essential practices for the attainment of discipline. But I have not yet mentioned the salutariness of silence as desirable in the preliminary stages. Silence is invariably associated with power. A silent man is one who has his emotions under his control. Silence acts on the finer aspects of one's psychological nature, and helps one to achieve his ends.

In general, nothing should be omitted to make the mind tranquil. It should be made as blank as a white sheet of paper. Then only will it be fit to receive perfect and permanent impressions.

In Hatha Yoga the mind is controlled by "Hatham," or violence. It is called the heroic method, and it brings

Consciousness

results in a short time. Here the mind is controlled through Prana (breath), the process being called Pranayama, or control of the Prana. Pranayama brings positive control over the mind, since the mind and breath are bound together, and by this practice the brain can be made insensible without being conscious of it. What appears to be sleep is really wakefulness in this art.

There are three obstacles to mental control: (1) Mental inertia, or laziness; (2) Distraction, a turning of the mind to irrelevant things; (3) Passions, impeding the mind's function by lust, and other desires.

When the mind is liberated from these, it becomes as motionless as a candle flame which is sheltered from all movement of the air. This is perfect meditation. When the mind is drowsy it should be promptly aroused. When it is distracted it should be made quiescent by turning it away from the object of the senses. When it is affected by passion, an effort should be made to banish the intruder. When it is still, it must not be disturbed. First there is a suppression of the agitation of the mind, followed by a cessation of the function of the mind as subject and object. When this stage is reached there comes the knowledge of the past and the future, a comprehension of the meaning of all Nature and its phenomena, a true realization of the Self.

4

The mind is the seat of appetites, sorrow, and infatuation, the fruit of which is either pleasure or pain. The Philosophy of Yoga dispenses with all such impediments to wisdom and true achievement. It removes all false notions of what life is, and it helps the disciple to gain control over all bodily passion. After this, it operates to develop the latent powers of the mind, to encourage the revelation of those powers and attributes, under specific conditions essential to this. Application and concentration are at the root of all success, whether worldly or spiritual. There are two tendencies ever present in the mind: one to excitement, the other to checking excitement. When one of these tendencies is defeated or suppressed, the other tendency grows more powerful.

Under this system the mind has five states:

1. Rajaguna. In this state it is restless, and roaming in all directions.
2. Tamaguna. In this state the wicked acts prompted by lust, anger, and the like appear to be proper to the mind.
3. Sattwaguna. In this state the mind is withdrawn toward various delights and forms of enjoyment.
4. Samadhi. In this state the mind is withdrawn from all objects other than that upon which it is centred.
5. Supreme Bliss. When the mind has reached the state of Samadhi it lets go its hold on all external objects and becomes dissolved in the source of its origin. In this state the disciple establishes his identity with the source of his Being.

The disciple first trains himself to make his mind vacant, so as to liberate it from all excitement, and to prepare it to receive that which the will imposes upon it. The will-power becomes master, and the mind works unaffected by its native impulses. This is the highest state of mental culture, in which man forgets the Self and acts for the realization of his highest duty. In the course of mental concentration the will-power is wholly immersed in the object of meditation, and gradually becomes identified with the object on which the disciple is concentrating. The closer the union between him and the object, the lesser will be the effort, and the mind will ultimately be reduced to a state of inaction.

The four stages in mental development are:

1. Abstraction. This consists in holding back the senses from their several objects.
2. Concentration. This is the fixing of the mind on any object.
3. Contemplation. This is the continued function of the mind upon an object, an even current of thought

undisturbed by other thoughts apart from the object upon which the mind has been placed.

4. Meditation. This is the resting of the mind on one thing, with all distinctions submerged, i.e., all distinctions between subject and object have vanished, and only pure thought remains. It is the realization of the thing contemplated.

Dhyana consists of a progressive state of consciousness, beginning with analysis, then reflection, which is a blissful state of consciousness; and proceeding to ecstasy, which comes into being when the apparent physical sensation of the former state gradually merges in the fourth state of cessation, which presents itself in a suspended condition and yields to complete concentration.

The Samadhi stage means that Uddiyana, Jalandhara, and Mulabundha have been accomplished, so that Prana Wayu (vital breath) has no other place to go but into the Sushumna. Prana Wayu has thus become suspended in one place, and can be taken up into the Thousand-Petalled Lotus in the Head. Ida, Pingala, and Sushumna are the three main Nadis (passages for nervous energy), which I have already described. Jalandhara and Mulabundha are two Mudras (bodily positions) which must be performed when practising Uddiyana, which is the first Yogic practice I have described. I will furnish further details later.

In contemplation there is a flow of mental activity, moulded into the form of the object of meditation, unimpeded by any other function. It is the flow of the thinking principle based upon steadiness in a particular place. Pure contemplation, which is Samadhi, a primordial state of mind, consists of being free from all ideas of the object and the contemplator. The meditator, having fixed his mind on Spirit, is oblivious of everything internal and external. Samadhi is the final stage of meditation. The Swamaji illustrated the idea with the following simile. A man afloat on a river passively submits to the current which bears him along smoothly. But let him once grasp at an object in the water, and the tranquillity of his motion is broken. In a like manner, thought formation arrests the natural flow of consciousness. By abiding in the mood of non-thought formation, Samadhi is attained.

This intense vividness is not a state of nothingness, but a void of unobstructed ecstatic blissfulness, consciousness itself as distinct from the knowing faculty by which it cognizes or knows itself to be. It is a void like a cloudless sky, an immutable light inseparable from the Great Body of Radiance, having no birth, no death, an eternal condition of boundless light. During ecstatic vision the Yogi sees the unevolved Self, free from all plurality, presented before the mind of the Higher Self. Those who contemplate Nature or God are interblended with it. They have passed through this state of Maya (unreality) and arrived at the Great Principle. This is not possible in the case of meditation. Abstract meditation has been called supportless meditation, because when it has been attained, all else has been completely destroyed; therefore, the Yogi is called unseeded. Such a mind has no further need of a physical body.

5

While in solitude, without any work to occupy one, the difficulty is to repress systematically all worldly thoughts and all the old familiar longings, a difficulty all the greater because the neophyte has toiled hard and long, apparently without result. It may seem to him as if he had made no progress whatsoever, and he may be almost inclined to give up in despair, when suddenly, he knows not why or how, his difficulty has disappeared and the seemingly impossible has become an accomplished fact.

There is no hard-and-fast rule as to what is to be done to achieve concentration and meditation. Exercises and detachment are to be used to the extent of one's power. One should never go to extremes, never go beyond the

Consciousness

point which is called "enough." An over-eager, over-hasty condition of the mind is hostile to success in concentration of mind. Proper food, Pranayama, and a suitable environment can do much to allay the hyper-excitement of the nerve centres.

Concentration is that state in which the mind is made to regulate the thinking processes, to direct thought to a single point. The practice (Abhyasa) of concentration is the repeated effort of holding Chitta in its unmanifested state, in a firm position, regardless of the end in view, uninterruptedly, over a long period of time. The idea is for the mind to retain a thought for the period of four minutes, without any effort on the part of the subject. This is the primary state of concentration. All thought movements (Writtis) then become coloured with this one thought or idea. In this state the mind is prevented from wandering. The processes of the mind are, at first, to form a taste, then a liking, then a desire, followed by a habit which develops into an instinct. These successive stages are subtly stamped upon the Chitta, forming potential values that are our Karma, causes of future desires, as the environment becomes fertile to the Chitta's expression. The root meaning of Chitta is that which gives the first ideation of things, the cause of causes, feeling as such. It is the waves on this feeling consciousness caused by thought-forms that give rise to differentiation (a world of desire). Its function is that of contemplation, whereby the mind forms for itself the object of its thought and dwells thereon. It is for this reason that it is also referred to as the Thinking Principle.

Chitta is the world of feeling, the ultimate reduction of everything to its seed, the seat of intelligence. As the space within the walls of a home constitutes the home, and not the walls, so is Chitta, the world of feeling, equivalent to the space that constitutes the home. It is that nothingness which counts for all things. In the case of the ordinary mind, Chitta becomes as restless as a wind-blown sea; the purpose of Yoga is to still this wind, so that the Chitta may become fixed and its Writti become a perfect reflection of undifferentiated existence, a reflection of the True Self. In deep sleep, all Writtis are submerged in their seat and become undifferentiated. Chitta can go anywhere, yet it is bound to the body. It is constantly running to all things, and it must be held in check; if it is allowed to run loose, Nirvana can never be attained.

If the action of the mind is suspended, the Chitta will dwell in the full knowledge of itself. Hence, the breath must be controlled, in order that Chitta may have a better channel through which to express itself. The waves of the Chitta, caused by thought forms, are called Writtis. The effect of all concentration is to colour the Writtis with the thing concentrated upon. These Writtis have to be stilled, made calm. A concentrated Writti is equal to about four minutes, and is called intentional Writti: for intention has been put behind it.

Chitta and Prana are very closely united. It is Karma that builds Chitta, and is its very substance. For perfect concentration, the Chitta must be permeated with Light and Truth. Concentration of the mind may be effected by pondering upon anything that one approves, by fixing the attention upon some object cognizable through the senses, as a point, a light (gross or subtle), space, a holy person, the tip of the nose, the centre of the tongue, Kundalini, the heart, the fire centre (navel), between the eyebrows, etc. The mind, having a predilection for forms, can be easily fixed on some form. Thus is it trained to fix itself on any chosen form, and it must be brought back to the object whenever it happens to stray from it. There will be a saving of energy if the object chosen for concentration be suited to the particular individual. A teacher with proper experience would be the best guide for this course.

To facilitate concentration, one may dwell on knowledge that presents itself in transition from the waking state to sleep; this transition is a natural one to a Yogi.

When passing from the wakeful state, the mind traverses a zero point attended by dreams when the mind is untrained. This zero point is an intermediate state between waking and sleeping, a comatose state, a state of natural concentration in which are retained the things impressed on it by training. When one dreams all night long, the conscious state is not fully submerged in the unconscious, and one remains at the threshold, some of the wakeful consciousness still diffused in the organs of sense. If the sensorium is witness to the dreams, they will be remembered; if the intelligence is witness, there will remain but a brief memory of them.

6

We should concentrate upon the thing which is most worth while to us, and review it until it acts as an obsession, or until we are conscious of the idea in all its detail. When we have done this several times, associated ideas will attach themselves to the central idea " I can do it," and will be supported by a substantial memory of having done something similar. Inferential memory compares everything. The triumphant memory testifies to what the senses have done in the past. The memory takes things from the senses. It is constantly on the watch. Without the phenomena of memory, we cannot have confidence. This confidence is not merely on the mental side, but it also comes from the already known past, having done certain things on the muscular side. Without this confidence, we cannot possess surety, or resolution necessary for accomplishment. It images the direct outcome of our memories. By way of memory the concrete is always translated into the abstract, and the abstract may be translated into the concrete. The concrete is limited by time and space, while the abstract is limited only by time.

Our memory is equal to our inclination to thought, and is the measure of the intensity of thought. All impressions are magnified or diminished by the degree of our attention. Memory also depends upon the quality of the body, which is the instrument of its action. When the physical channels are imperfect, the memory is affected and corrupted. On the other hand, absence of memory is often due to a lack of desire to project the memory into the future; that is, we would like to remember, or have an inclination for future memory, but no desire to make it a reality in the present.

The will, a source of abstract energy, is the work of intelligence. It is discrimination, the directing power. It is within the power of the will to enforce or inhibit unfavourable tendencies. To hold a mental concept before the mind in the absence of the corresponding object, to reproduce, to modify and to combine materials furnished, are all functions within the power of the will. Attention plays a significant part in concentration, for it forms the basis of the will. Properly directed towards the internal world with the object of introspection, it functions in the analysis of the mind and illumines all facts. It is through the power of attention that the mind carries on its activities.

Fixation and one-pointedness of attention induce a sort of trance and exultation of the mental faculties. To induce this trance state, selective attention is used. This may be called the spotlight of the intellect, for one cultivates the power of visualization, and of feeling, with which come greater discrimination, greater comprehension, greater ability. By artificially intensifying the natural mental processes, the mind concentrates itself readily and wholly upon the object of its attention at the expense of what is a general and many-sided alertness and awareness. If we want an idea in the world of thought, we should translate it from the world of feeling. Likewise, if we have a strong emotion as the result of some contact of the senses, we should translate it into the world of thought. This will facilitate internal growth.

7

Thus we talked all night. Then came the dawn. Since there were many things to attend to before the evening train left, we begged leave to decline the Swamaji's invitation to partake of a little food before departure.

It was an inspiring morning. I felt sensible of the urge of life, and from my high point of exultation it was difficult to return to reality. It was as if I had come from another world, the world I had so often dreamed of; I could scarcely believe that what I had so ardently wished for had actually come to pass. I was living the life I had wanted.

But few words were exchanged between my Tantrik friend and myself as our boat silently glided along with the current of the stream to the rhythm of oars lapping on the water. I passed the moments in a sort of trance imposed on me by the experience of the night. The answers to my questions were rapidly being given me. And now it was up to me to find the way to make the thought substance of that experience a part of me, a part of my second nature. The way would come. I felt confident of that.

We landed in the city amidst the great throngs which come to the banks of India's sacred river to worship and to wash away their sins each morning. As we drove back to my residence, we wove our way in and out, through the endless crowds of devotees carrying their small brass jugs filled with holy water. Others who had already attended their morning Puja (worship) were driving their herds of cows and goats through the streets; yet others were bringing their products to the market in wobbly carts drawn by trudging water buffaloes. The sun had just risen above the horizon, and the streets were beginning to steam, and the air was rapidly growing thick and slimy. The beggars were at their posts; the lepers were holding out their rotting arms, imploring for morning alms.

But little time was wasted in throwing the few things together that were still unpacked. I hurried to the telegraph office. Giving my cables to the Babu (clerk), I asked him how much it would be to send a cable to New York City, and another to Arizona. I had by now grown somewhat familiar with the Indian way of doing things, so I was not particularly disturbed when the Babu did not show up for about half an hour. I knew that he was looking through the regulations to assist me. At last, looking up from a large book, he threw out his chest and strolled over to the window. There was no such place as New York City, he announced. Forgetting my Eastern teachings, I felt like committing murder. My rage soon brought several assistants to his rescue; after I had quieted down I again explained the simple nature of my quest. They disappeared, and presently returned with the same answer: there was no such place as New York City. I demanded the book, and pointed out what I wanted in ten seconds. They said that I was inaccurate, for the regulations read New York, New York, and not New York City. To their chagrin, I insisted, however, that that was the place where my cable was going.

Now I was beginning to have dubious feelings about what might happen to Arizona. And, indeed, after again consulting their book, they returned with the information that there was no such place. I was driven to draw a map of Arizona, indicating that it was almost as big as their country. That settled them for a while, but they returned with the question: did I want Arizona in Canada, in South America, or in the United States? I must confess that this was something new to me; I had never suspected that there could be an Arizona other than the large state I knew. In just a little less than an hour and a half we had managed to determine the amount of postage required. I do not exaggerate. I still had to purchase my stamps, which is the way you pay for cables. These are bought at another window and pasted on the cable, which is turned in at the original window of inquiry. The individual who sold them was not there. It seems it was teatime, or some other such rest period, with which business must not be allowed to interfere. Soon, however, he appeared; and it took him just about fifteen minutes to count out the stamps and make out the change. What a relief it was, immediately afterwards, to walk into the American Express office and have one say in about ten seconds that he would see to it that everything was taken care of according to my instructions. I should have gone there in the first place, but I was trying to get the feel of the country by looking for local colour. I fear that all the colour was being exhibited by me (red, I imagine) by my constant state of rage, which presented such a violent contrast to the tranquil state of mind I was instructed to induce. Now I understood what the Swamaji meant when he said that one's environment so often offered the greatest obstacle on the way to Eternal Truth.

In India it is wise to have everything finished up a day ahead of time; there is no such thing as rushing through. To taste of the country's sleeping consciousness, it is necessary to learn the art of leisure and relaxation, so difficult for an American. Our breakneck speed has no validity in that land. External matters are of no particular importance. They must be attended to, of course; but they can wait, so why hurry? A little of this attitude wouldn't hurt us if we practised it at home.

My Tantrik friend accompanied me to the railway station, since it was to be my first experience of taking an Indian train. I arrived at a scene not so unlike those of our own stations. The coolie porters clamoured round me to carry my endless packages at an anna a package. The American habit of using large trunks is not popular here. I emulated the English traveller's custom of carrying fifteen or twenty small parcels without exhibiting the least embarrassment. I let the coolies carry everything but my fountain pen and my Leica. On entering the waiting-room I was surprised to find countless hundreds of natives, wrapped in white cloth, all squatting on the floor, surrounded by their humble possessions.

When the train pulled in, the platform was comparable to a beehive. With the help of many coolies and my friend, I managed to get aboard, and found myself cheerfully crowded in a compartment with seven native passengers. Along with all of one's luggage, it is necessary to carry one's own bedding. Since each of us had about ten more bundles than was convenient, it was something of a problem how to dispose of our belongings. We managed somehow by storing away most of them in the upper berths, permitting us to stretch out a little during the night on the narrow, hard, leather-padded benches along the walls.

At this early period of my visit to India, I was not yet sufficiently acquainted with its people to differentiate between them. The common run of them all looked pretty much alike to me. It was only a question of one being thin and another being a little thinner. Luckily for me, considering the limited space offered by the compartment, my companions were mostly on the very thin side. They were attired in their cool and comfortable dhotis, while I was sweltering in my sopping tropical linens. The fans were going full blast, and I was still mopping my brow when the train pulled out of the sticky station. I was off.

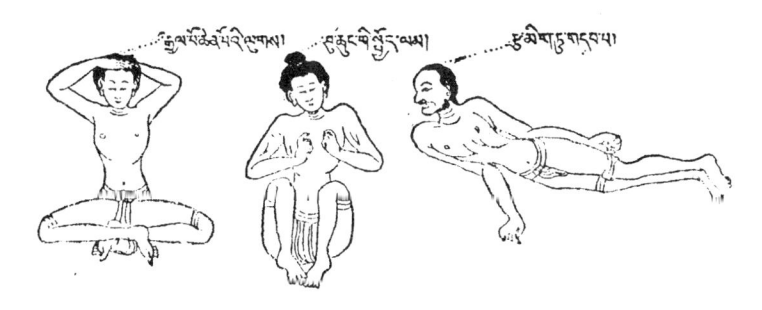

CHAPTER X

SIGHTS AND EXPERIENCES IN INDIA

I

IT may seem odd that I should begin this chapter with some account of my return to Calcutta after long months of travel across the length and breadth of the strange land. Yet this is not so odd when you take into consideration the main object of my journey and the fact that, from my own point of view, it is not the journey itself day by day, but the journey seen in perspective that counts for anything in this narrative of spiritual experience in which, directly and indirectly, Yoga and the quest of Yoga play a significant part.

I was greeted on my early morning arrival by countless crows which crowd the Calcutta air, filling it with their raucous cries. I was glad to be back. Happy in the knowledge that it is never too early to visit a friend in India, I promptly set out for my Tantrik friend's home, only to be informed that he had gone to his place in the hills. The Swamaji, too, had fled to his jungle hermitage. Indeed, I found that all of my friends in the city had left town shortly after my departure and had not yet returned. I had promised to get into prompt touch with my Tantrik friend upon my return; so without much ado I repacked and was soon on my way to his retreat.

It was a warm welcome that I received there. Few people in the world can surpass the Indians in hospitality. They always make you feel as if you were one of the family, and the favourite one at that. It did my heart good to feel the bond of such friendship, and we lost no time in taking up the thread where we left off.

In short, we plunged into a review of my journey. It had its high and its low spots, its comforts and discomforts, its depressions and exultations, and I had met all sorts of persons, ranging from Rajas to Beggars, Kavirajas to Magicians, Scholars to Students, Saints to Sadus. I saw all the glories of India: Allahabad, Benares, Agra, Delhi, Lahore, Srinagar in Kashmir, Peshwar, the Kyber, Uddipur, Bombay, Hyderabad, Mysore, Bangalore, Madras, Madura, Trichinopoly, and then a tour of Ceylon. I had missed nothing, from broad ways to back alleys; I visited palaces, forts, museums, colleges, libraries, temples, ashrams, ghats, and shrines galore. I had learned the significance of the statement that India is steeped in the mire of ignorance, but that it is also the womb of all philosophy. All that is true.

We talked far into the night. I was reliving my journey, reliving it in the light of a new wisdom that comes after the event and of analysis that comes of two minds working together to glean the grain from the chaff.

2

My Tantrik friend asked me as to what I thought was the most memorable experience of my journey. I could not determine that at the moment, and I laughingly countered that I surely knew which experience was the most embarrassing. And I proceeded to relate it.

I had come to India, I said, to learn its teachings and not primarily to see its sights. Being an American, the last thing that ever entered my mind was to carry a " white tie " with me; indeed, it was only by chance that I had even a dinner jacket. By a piece of good fortune I arrived at Mysore during the important religious festival, the Dasara, that lasts ten days and includes the great Durbar. I was the guest of the Prime Minister of the State, to whom I had a letter of introduction from mutual friends in America. He sent me an invitation from the Maharajah to attend the Durbar. Here was my opportunity to be presented to one of the most famed Maharajahs of India. As a child I vividly pictured in the passing clouds all the pomp and pageantry of King Arthur's Court. And here a twentieth-century fairy tale was going to come true for me. It is not every one that gets the chance to be presented to India's most celebrated Maharajah.

On examining the engraved invitation, I noticed its very formal character, and read that all officers were to come in uniform, wearing all their medals of honour. The latter stipulation gave me no trouble, as I possessed neither a uniform nor medals; and the card did not mention any tails. After all, I was travelling around the world, and it could scarcely be expected that I should provide myself with all the trappings of an ultra-sophisticated life. At all events, I did possess a dinner jacket, and as I groomed myself in it I felt that I was more than presentable, it never having occurred to me in that moment that there is such a thing as the pride that goeth before the fall. As I was a guest of the State, a car was provided by the Prime Minister to fetch me to the spectacle. Indeed, no effort was spared to see to my every need, with the possible exception of a "white tie."

The Durbar was to be held at eight, and I asked that the car be sent to me much earlier so as to permit me to look around a bit on my arrival, as I counted on the event to be one of the richest treats of my life. The palace grounds were surrounded by a high wall with a beautiful arched entrance all illuminated by electricity, which by no means obscured the magnificence of the marble palace that was silhouetted against the blackness of the night, its vast shape outlined by a myriad of sparkling electric light bulbs. As I stepped from the car at the entrance of the long arcade which led into the majestic palace, two attendants, who were Knights of the Court, approached me and mentioned the fact that my coat was a trifle short. Looking back over my shoulder, and glancing down at my heels, I replied that that was the way it was cut. Ignorant as they were of my identity, it would have been embarrassing for them to pursue the subject; they knew that if everything was not in order I would be stopped by someone else at the entrance. With my head high, and my shoulders at attention, I sauntered along with all the decorum I could muster, taking in everything and everybody; for the Knights of England were arriving with their Ladies, a spectacle which makes the Easter parade look like a barmaids' holiday.

I cautiously followed a large group and was lost to the eye of the doorman. Once inside, the ladies and gentlemen left to remove their wraps, and I found myself standing alone in the middle of a beautifully decorated vestibule. I overheard some one to the effect that the Durbar Hall was upstairs. As I began my ascent another set of attendants followed me with the admonition that my coat was too short. I fully agreed with them, and continued my ascent. Presently I found myself in the midst of the most dazzling sight that I had beheld in many a day—the great Durbar Hall. It was an immense hall with a high scalloped ceiling inlaid with glittering stones; with each step you took the colours changed, giving the sense of a richly hued kaleidoscope. And immediately in front of the carved columns which held up the roof was the jewelled throne of the Maharajah. I was overcome with it all as if I had actually found myself in King Arthur's Court.

Preoccupied as I was with the details of the resplendent grandeur and with the moving spectacle of Lords and Knights and Ladies, I was hardly aware of the passage of time. Soon, however, every one began to fall in line. The Maharajah was approaching. My own body was in line, but my head was very much out of order; for I was trying to look in all directions at once without losing my place, which I had skilfully managed to obtain so as to be in a position of vantage when his Highnesss entered. Just as he came into the great hall, a couple of attendants interrupted my observations of his jewelled crown and stately robes. This time they said: "Sir, you are not wearing a 'white tie' this evening." Again I readily agreed. I tried to shake them off, but they insisted that there was a regrettable formality: no one was permitted to march before his Highness without a "white tie." So I was escorted behind the forming line and led to a chair, where I might sit and watch the entertainment which was to take place in the large amphitheatre just below us. The arrangement of our seats was very much like that in a large covered grandstand. I was particularly interested in the people, because, though excellent, the entertainment was of a modern nature.

Lost in reverie, the time flew by. The moment for departure arrived. Every one was to march past in front of his Highness, who was to present a corsage to each of the Ladies. Now I felt that my opportunity had at last arrived, but my attached friends, the two attendants, had other plans for me. They insisted on escorting me out of danger. And so once more I found myself among the columns; here I was left to roam at large, a cynosure for the eyes of the Lords and Knights and Ladies, who glimpsed at me curiously out of the corners of their eyes and whispered I knew not what sort of comments.

And, again, one of my attendants headed towards me. This time, in a very polite manner, he asked whose guest I was. The Maharajah's, said I. Without a further word he went to the Prime Minister, whose presence I had avoided because I had seen how busy he was. He must have assured the attendant that I was an honoured guest, for from that instant I became the victim of the most assiduous attention. But the Durbar was over, and I had not been presented.

My Tantrik friend then impressed upon me that in the practice of Yoga one must always be prepared outwardly, as well as inwardly, to meet the world in which one lives.

So I learned that even a Yogi needs a "white tie"!

3

The next morning at breakfast my host inquired about the teachers and the holy men I had met. There was time enough to touch only on the high spots.

At Benares I had seen countless thousands of faithful worshippers who go each morning to the ghats on the banks of the sacred Ganges to wash away their sins. Many of them wait to die here, for the devotee feels that it is auspicious to die on the banks of the sacred river, and they come from all corners of India when they feel that their hour is near. We both agreed as to the filth and folly of the procedure, which is but an empty form. Sins are washed away from within. And this was but a symbol.

At Delhi I had learned what was being done to revive the ancient native system of medicine as taught and practised by the Kavirajas (native doctors), who have gained their knowledge by word of mouth from their ancestors as it has been passed along century after century. I was shown how some of their medicines were prepared from diamonds, gold, pearls, sandalwood, etc. I had even tasted of them. The art of preparing mercury, so that it can be taken by the Yogi during his training, has been lost for centuries, but you can still purchase mercury to be used for medicinal purposes if you care to take it. Indeed, you can find almost any medicine you want.

In Bombay I met several people who are known to the public by their writings. Two visits which I enjoyed were to the authors of two books on Yoga. One was a visit to S'rimat Kuvalayananda at his Ashrama at Lonavla, near Bombay, where Doctor Kovoor T. Behanan had spent two years studying while he gathered material for his *Scientific Evaluation of Yoga* for his Doctorate degree at Yale University. I had studied with considerable care the journals which S'rimat Kuvalayananda had published on the Asanas and Pranayama. When he learned of my interests and studies, he was anxious to do everything in his power to further my own investigations. He told me of a famed Holy Man in Hyderabad whom he thought I should like to meet. Gurus vary just as pupils do ; each has his own particular method, suited better to one pupil than another, so I wanted to meet as many as possible in order to broaden my knowledge. In any event, I was determined to try to find him, not to permit any opportunity to pass me by.

Another visit was to Mr. Vasant G. Rele, of Bombay, author of *The Mysterious Kundalini*. Having for many years studied the works of Sir John Woodruffe (Arthur Avalon), who has provided us with our most authoritative translation of many of the Tantrik doctrines which hold Kundalini to be the Life Force of Man, I was particularly interested in meeting Doctor Rele, who had a theory of his own on this mysterious force, which he associated with the glandular system of the body, thereby abolishing the mystery of the " Coiled Serpent " that is believed to be within us. He took issue with some of the theories propounded by Arthur Avalon in his book entitled *Serpent Power*. I listened to his views, all the more as I knew that the time was approaching when I should have to make an intense study of the theory of this doctrine with my Tantrik friend.

I had been instructed many years ago to study everything and accept nothing, for there would be constant change as I continued to grow. Never was I to become crystallized in static understanding. There were always deeper depths ahead, and the prerequisite for solving them was an open mind. So I merely asked endless questions and listened with a receptive mind to another set of settled answers. The one thing most apparent during my investigations was that every one with whom I talked had the ultimate answer. The others, surely, must have been in the wrong. Thus I continued filling my basket with plucked finalities from the tottering trees of prejudice.

In Bombay, as well as in other centres, I met many others who were scholarly versed in the teachings of

Yoga. It was easy enough to find those who could demonstrate all of Yoga's esoteric teachings. But those who possessed its esoteric knowledge were always far removed from the main highways, and known only to small groups of friends whose high regard for their noble pursuit in this life kept them from revealing to the public where they lived.

4

On leaving Bombay, I promptly set out to find the Holy Man of Hyderabad. I soon learned that my man was now living in Madras; so, without losing a moment, I was off again. On reaching Madras, I had the task before me of discovering his address. I drove in a taxi-cab from street to street, from corner to corner. Fortunately I ran into someone who knew of him, and when I finally found his place, it was only to discover that he was away; no one knew how long he would be gone. He was on a pilgrimage. This might last a day or a lifetime. As I continued my way to Ceylon, I kept on in vain asking about him; he had a reputation throughout most of South India. On my return to Madras, I again went to the place where I had found his friends during my earlier visit. They had moved, and no one knew anything about them. Then I began to comb the bookshops and the libraries in an effort to find some of his publications; but as he wrote in his native tongue it didn't help me much, though I continued my search. I did finally discover the name of his publishers. On visiting them, they told me that the Holy Man had gone to Mysore. So I was off again, only to be redirected back to Bangalore, where I was graciously received by Shri Paramahamta Sachitananda Yogiswarar in his modest sanctuary, where he pursued his studies in order that he might illuminate the way for the spiritual growth of his people.

He was a man of thin frame, with a large stomach. His long white hair, folding in with his uncut beard, gracefully dropped over his shoulders and chest. Though he was in his late sixties, he was still very vigorous. Every syllable he spoke was clipped with vitality. His eyes sparkled as they could only in one who is clean within. They glistened with a radiance of inner wealth in the understanding of life. His entire existence had been devoted to his spiritual development. Now he was dedicating the remainder of his days to the help of others. His knowledge of native teachings was extensive as well as profound, and he had worked for years on the art of Pranayama, control of the breath. In order to reveal to me his development of this art, he brought out pictures of himself taken when he was sitting on top of the water teaching a group of disciples. From him I learned another technique of the art of Pranayama. This being virtually the Key to Yoga, I was ever trying to learn more about it ; for I knew that this was going to be the path I should have to follow when again the time came for me to enter the harness of discipline.

5

My host being one of the few persons I had met who held an open mind and was always eager to gain further knowledge from the experience of others, asked me to repeat the technique as it had been given me by the Holy Man.

The technique taught by the Holy Man was of the common-run knowledge ; so my Tantrik friend proceeded to reveal to me a special technique known only to a few men who have accomplished things and who are not content with anything less than the shortest and most heroic means of attaining their ambition.

I was told that this was a special technique for the benefit of those who had already been disciples for some time and were proficient in the important methods of purification—Dhauti, Neti, Basti, Nauli, Trataka, and Kapalabhati—and had perfected all the necessary Asanas and Mudras. In other words, it was only for the well trained. He had pointed out that there were a great many methods of Pranayama, and that different practitioners stressed different ones. He added that for the most part they were all very slow in developing the individual; that some of them, indeed, had no value whatsoever. It was becoming obvious that it behoved the student to know almost as much as the teacher if he was to discriminate between the helpful method and one that was wholly futile. The special technique was substantially as follows:

After taking your seat in Siddhasana or Padmasana, take about four mouthfuls of cool sweet water and bring the body to an erect position with the head in a restful position; then close the mouth and keep the teeth firmly pressed together. After closing the eyes, focus them at the tip of the nose and observe your breathing. Now exhale the breath from the lungs, with effort, clearing out every vestige of air. This is possible by three final exclamations of " UH ! ", a sort of pig-like grunt. Next place the thumb of the right hand on the right nostril with the ring and little fingers of the same hand on the left nostril; then, closing the right nostril, inhale to capacity through the left one. There is no need to pack the air in. After you have filled the lungs, swallow as though you were swallowing saliva, dropping the chin deep into the small pocket at the base of the neck (this is called Jalandhara) and suspend breathing. The hands may now be returned to the knees or kept in that position. While suspending the breath, count slowly up to fifty, or to whatever number happens to be your comfortable limit. You are always cautioned never to suspend the breath to the point of gasping for air. When a reasonable limit has been reached, you close the left nostril, allowing the air to escape with restraint through the right nostril to a distance of some four inches. This is to be done until the tension in the lungs has been reduced a trifle; then immediately inhale through the right nostril in order to fill the lungs again; then reverse the process through the left nostril. After taking the air in again through the left nostril, let it out once more, as before, through the right. This process of short breathing is to be kept up until you can no longer hold the breath. The lungs are then to be slowly emptied until every vestige of air is gone from them, after which normal breathing may be resumed. A period of rest is to be taken, and then the same technique repeated. While resting it is wise to fix the mind and not allow it any action. This is known as Unmani—no mind. The mouth should be kept tightly closed during each round. The above process is counted as a single round of Pranayama.

In the beginning the breath will naturally tend to escape more completely on each short breath, but this must be controlled after the manner described. At no time must the breath be allowed to escape quickly from the lungs, permitting them to relax completely. After the rest period, the process should be repeated. This time the breath should be taken through the right nostril. The practice of alternating from one nostril to the other should be followed, even during the period of short-breathing. This period may be kept up for some five minutes after one has practised it for a time. After each round, one is to sit quietly with the hands resting on the knees or thigh, at the same time keeping the mind a blank, and the eyes are fixed between the eyebrows.

When the practice has been developed to the point that it can be properly performed with comfort, the second round is altered. After the rest period of the first round, you are to begin to fill the lungs through the right nostril, allowing only four inches of air to enter at this nostril; then shift to the left, then to the right, and so on, until the lungs have been completely filled, the last breath being taken through the right nostril. After swallowing, suspend the breath for the same number of counts as before; then start the short-breathing until your power of restraint is gone. The lungs are then to be slowly and completely emptied by the utterance of the sound "UH" (as already explained), and the abdomen is to be pressed in with each sound. Only the surface tension is to be allowed to escape in this act of short-breathing, the air being allowed to flow down about four inches from the nostril. This is very important. The instinct is to allow the entire quantity of air to rush out; this must be checked. The inhalation and exhalation must be accomplished slowly. The duration of the Kumbhaka (suspension) should never be permitted to exceed one's reasonable limitations. One must never go to an extreme. The length of time for this suspension should be increased slowly, and only after each practice period has been developed to a reasonable state of perfection. One deals with power here, so every care should be taken to develop it gradually and slowly.

The diet must be considered from the point of view of the individual. His requirements will vary according to his bodily condition. A sufficient quantity of milk and clarified butter is desirable; in the beginning, however, the Ghee (clarified butter) should be taken with some caution. Thought should be given to one's power of digestion and assimilation. Three meals a day may be taken at the start, if only one fourth of the stomach is filled at the morning meal, three fourths at the midday meal, and one half a stomachful in the evening. Black pepper and ginger may be taken, in order to aid the digestion and warm the stomach. A little of something sour may be taken to flavour the food, when needed. Wheat, rice, green gram (luctow), Ghee, and milk may be used among the staple food products, in small quantities. Pure cane sugar or honey may be used to sweeten things. As time goes on, the diet must be reduced to a fixed standard and is to consist almost wholly of fluids. This cannot and should not be done at the start, as it will lead to disastrous results. A period of thirty minutes must elapse after a practice before food is taken; a small glass of milk, however, may be taken immediately.

As for sexual intercourse, one may indulge twice a month without detriment, but one must be cautious and conserve the vital fluid to the utmost.

Sights and Experiences in India

To seek to master the breath in a hurry is to court disaster. It is only after a lapse of time, after much experience, after a slow development of one's capacity, that there is an accretion of power from the art of Pranayama. The pupil may begin by doing three practices a day: morning, noon, and evening. He must exercise caution and not exceed his capacity at the moment; he must not reach the point where his energies are exhausted. The practice must be regular, have its appointed time; results will be apparent in the long run. Eventually the Prana (breath) will yield its great tension in the body, and the student will discover that he can hold it with ease. At the beginning, after practice, the nerves may be a little trying, and one may suffer slight convulsions. There is no need for anxiety about this if one will but adhere to a good portion of wheat, or barley, or rich milk and some Ghee at meals. The nervous feeling will pass off in due course. At the beginning, too, the perspiration will flow rather freely. This bodily dampness, however, should not be wiped off, but massaged into the body, as though one were taking an oil bath.

It will be found that fifty counts (seconds) of Kumbhaka are quite sufficient at the start; it is advisable to hold to this for two months. When this is accomplished with ease, the number of counts may be increased to seventy-five or more. There is no need to be alarmed over any pain that develops; within two months or so there will be no indication of it. The pain should be used as a measuring rod, and the next step should be avoided until it has subsided.

When he has reached the point where he could do one hundred seconds of Kumbhaka, the student should exhale to the navel, then inhale this amount of breath immediately and repeat the Kumbhaka for another one hundred seconds, and then exhale again to the distance of the navel through the opposite nostril, promptly inhaling and repeating the Kumbhaka for one hundred counts. He is to repeat this until he has done the Kumbhaka one, two, three, four, or five times, which will be equal to a control over the breath for the same number of hundred-seconds: 100, 200, 300, 400, 500. He may then advance his Kumbhaka to 125 seconds, breathing alternately through the left and right nostrils, and finally through both nostrils simultaneously, and slowly increase the capacity to 150 to 200 seconds, or more, according to his development. The longer the Kumbhaka, the more freely the body will perspire, because the Kumbhaka increases the heat of the body. In order to mitigate this when it becomes too intense, the practice may be done in water, or one may massage the body from the top of the head to the feet with a mixture of almond milk, almond oil, with a little black pepper or ginger juice, saffron, and such articles as are cooling in their nature. Such balms should be left on the body for half an hour or more, in order that they may soak in freely. This should be done twice a week.

After the full Kumbhaka has been accomplished, the breath should be allowed to escape in small gusts, now through one nostril and then through the other, until the lungs have been deflated. Then inhale after the same fashion, taking the short breath to the navel previous to each Kumbhaka. The process is to be persisted in until the Kumbhaka has been done to a total of 1200 seconds. Gradually the process is increased until the student can suspend the breath for 3000 or 5000 seconds.

The air will remain in the lungs until about 4000 seconds of Kumbhaka has been reached; then it will try to force itself out of the lungs and seek to enter the alimentary canal. There will be experienced a sort of kicking back against the throat, as it tries to enter the œsophagus and the stomach. The Yogi aids this process by swallowing and pressing the chin into the hollow of the neck (Jalandhara Mudra). It will be discovered in this operation that the air encounters an obstruction in its downward movement which makes it rebound again to the throat; hence, you must maintain this chin lock and prevent the air from escaping. This process of rebounding will be encountered again and again throughout the entire course into and through the whole length of the alimentary track. When the air has reached the anus one should lock it (Mulabandha) by contracting the sphincters of the rectum and thereby prevent its escape. This operation will be attended with considerable pain at the start, but it will disappear with time, and the process will become quite natural and easy.

During the development of the practice the bowels will croak and the air will be felt moving from one side to the other below the navel. In order to prepare the way for the air to enter the alimentary canal, it is advisable to take about four mouthfuls of water just before starting Pranayama. At meals it will be likewise advantageous to consume a small quantity of barley, wheat, or rice, which is well soaked with Ghee in order to lubricate the channels and facilitate the entry of food into the stomach and bowels. The greater the capacity for Kumbhaka, the longer will the practitioner be free from hunger. This effect is due to the air circulating throughout the alimentary canal, and the process is called "Living on Air." When the individual has attained this stage, he can successfully reduce his diet to rich milk, Ghee, and a few sweet fruits and begin his practices on concentration and meditation.

Pranayama may be considered sufficiently developed when one can do Kumbhaka for five or six minutes. At this stage the Yogi may engage himself in training the mind for one-pointedness. The mind will soon become self-centred, no matter where it is placed, and one can then begin the awakening of Kundalini. In the event of the mind becoming restless during the period of meditation, it can be stilled by merely lowering the gaze and making relaxation the chief aim.

In order to accomplish the "Greater Kumbhaka," one should begin by closing the left nostril and inhaling through the right, and proceed with a Kumbhaka lasting 15,000 counts. Then one exhales through the right nostril and immediately inhales through the left, repeating the Kumbhaka for 15,000 counts. This process is to be repeated until one has done four such Pranayamas. Then one closes the right nostril and exhales through the left to a distance of four inches, inhaling the same quantity of air through the same nostril. It is permissible to allow the breath to play back and forth within the limits of that distance, but at all times the bulk of the air must be retained in the lungs, and the practice is to be finished off as indicated. It will be found that this method will yield a net Kumbhaka of 60,000 seconds.

In order to transcend the pale of relativity and conditional existence, so that one might enter into Union with the Universal Spirit and thereby secure Self-Forgetfulness by entering into a superconscious state of Self-Abstraction, it is necessary to begin by inhaling through the right nostril and to proceed with a Kumbhaka of 12,000 seconds. Afterwards the disciple must sit in concentration for ten minutes. He is to repeat the process, this time inhaling through the left nostril. Following with ten minutes of concentration, he must repeat the process, through both nostrils. It will not be long before all the senses of the body will cease their activity. Samadhi can be reached when the Kumbhaka is developed to 60,000 seconds. By doing it gradually, one should be able to control the breath for one and a half hours; then only will the psychic powers manifest themselves.

When one has been able to hold his breath for some 3000 to 5000 seconds, he will feel it permeating his entire body. There will be experienced a tingling and stinging sensation over the entire surface. This will disappear immediately on exhaling. One must do Kumbhaka without any fear and endure these experiences if any progress is to be made. And again it must be stressed that the diet must be very closely watched in order that the digestion remain in its best possible condition. It is essential to have the proper amount of oily food (Ghee), in order to keep the nerves soothed and the body properly lubricated.

It is well to bear in mind that the best time of the year for taking up the practice of Pranayama is in March and April or September and October. It is never to be commenced in the hot, cold, or rainy seasons. During the hot weather the Yogi uses the nights for his practice.

6

The breakfast hour had long passed, and it was time to begin the day. My Tantrik friend assured me that what he had related was one of the most important techniques on the practice of Pranayama. It is rarely that this method is imparted to another before he has experienced a long period of discipleship. It was evident, however, that the mere oral detailing of a practice was in no sense a full revelation of a technique. The guiding hand of a teacher was essential. Different obstacles usually arose with different individuals, and only he who knew the Law upon which all the Yogic techniques were based could help the pupil overcome his specific difficulty. The techniques of most of the Yogic practices were to be obtained in books, but it is uncomfortably true that even written instructions are insufficient. There is no correspondence course to Heaven.

Since it was my plan eventually to pass on these teachings to others in the West, my Tantrik friend pointed out the necessity of my learning the simplest forms. He promised to inform me at teatime some of the fundamentals of these; in the meantime he had his own studies to attend to, and I had mine.

I returned to my small whitewashed room with its simple furnishings consisting of a warped table and chair and a few nails on the wall on which to hang my clothes. I had still my bags to unpack and other things to do preliminary to taking up my studies. After a light lunch I welcomed a period of relaxation, as this was the first time I had come to a halt since leaving Bangalore. My mind wandered, speculating on the future. I experienced the growing feeling that my efforts were not in vain, that I was following a divinely directed urge, which troubled me every time that I stepped out of the predestined course. I was very much aware of the fact that I was becoming gorged with theory and information. I was growing increasingly restless with my desire to translate it all into action.

For the time being, however, I had to content myself with my studies and my daily period of " Silence," during which I indulged in introspection. I had become as devoted to this as a Hindu. I knew it was not for me to rush things. To prepare and to wait—this was my task. Somewhere, someone was watching me; when the hour came that I was ready, all the rest would follow. I reflected on the thought, that he who spends the longest period in preparation makes the greatest headway when the proper time comes, under the guidance of his Guru. I would be patient.

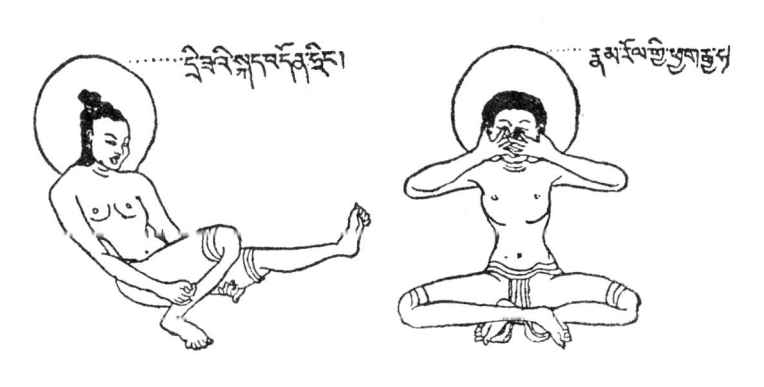

CHAPTER XI

MORE ABOUT THE SCIENCE OF BREATH

I

FOUR o'clock had arrived, and I went to the simple sitting-room of my friend. We disposed of ourselves comfortably on the floor. By sitting in this manner at all times, I was rapidly growing to find greater relaxation in it than in sitting on a chair. It had the extra advantage in that it stretched the limbs, so that when the time came for me to take up the Asanas, I would be able to master them in a relatively short time. I had always been quite limber; hence, I did not have to go through the period of intense discomfort that is the lot of most Westerners who have tried to accustom themselves to the ways of the Hindu at home. Scarcely had our tea been served when my friend began to instruct me.

Before it is possible for one fully to accomplish the art of Pranayama, it is imperative to inform oneself about the theory upon which it is based. Until one has perfected his Pranayama, however, it is next to impossible to make use of one's knowledge of the theory. Hence it was necessary for me to know something of the fundamentals before proceeding with my work.

In order to make greater headway with my practice of Pranayama when I took up the discipline, my friend was going to give me such material as would be helpful to my immediate needs. It is evident that the more I knew of the theory, the stronger would be my urge to become competent on the path of Yoga which results in definite victory. I realized that I was being instructed in such a manner that I would surely gain the goal for which I was striving.

First he related to me, in a general way, the theory of breath as expounded in the Tantrik work known as the Swarodaya.

No theory about the Life of the Universe is so simple, yet so grand and sufficient as the theory of Breath. Breath (Prana) is the inseparable power (Shakti) of God. It is the Supreme Power over all created things, the Life Principle of the Universe. It is the substratum of all cause and effect, which are held like beads on this thread of life. Shakti (power) is ever present in man. Breath (Prana) first came out of God. It is the breath of God which breathed forth the Universe and which in the end will be inhaled back to God. In its extent it is said to be as incomprehensible as the Ocean of Infinity. It is the mind of man which prevents him from becoming conscious of its presence.

The word Prana comes from the Sanskrit root "Pra," meaning First. "Na" means the smallest unit of force. Hence, Prana stands for First Breath. All action is nothing but a change in the phases of Prana.

In the science of Yoga, its function is the law of the existence of the Universe. It is brought into existence and kept in activity by the Sun itself. Its reflection in man is what gives birth to human breath. When it enters the individual it becomes divided into the ten functions of Wayu. Each of the ten functions has its own name: Prana, Apana, Samana, Udana, Vyana, Naga, Kurma, Krkara, Devadatta, and Dhanamjaya.

Prana, the Life Principle, is the dynamic or working force of man and of all living things. It is the power which supports the body and all its moving forces. It is the dwelling place of Jiva (soul). The Nadis (nerve channels) of the body are the tubes through which Prana moves.

2

This science of breath has its foundation in the control of Prana. It is of the highest importance to any student of Yoga. This is the most useful, comprehensive, and interesting branch of Yoga.

By the means of Prana, light is cast over all Name and Form. Therefore the wise will study the regulation of Prana if they desire to suspend the activity of the Mind and concentrate the will upon the achievement of Yoga.

The control of the breath leads to health, the growth of strength, energy, fine complexion, increased vitality, growth in the knowledge and extension of life. It is the breath that upholds the constituents of the body: blood, flesh, marrow, bone, etc. It creates all the movements in the body. It restrains the mind from undesirable objects and concentrates it solely upon desired ones. The functions of the ten senses of knowledge and action are dependent on it. It gives form to the embryo in the womb. It furnishes the evidence of the existence of life, since it is the cause of speech, touch, sound, and scent, and is the origin of joy and cheer. It excites the fires of the body and creates the heat which burns out all the impurities of the body; it pierces through all the ducts of the body, gross and delicate, disposing of all diseases.

The Vital Air or respiration is the manifestation of the Life Coil which draws atmospheric air from without into the system. It is what causes the forward and backward motions of the breath to the extent of eight to twelve inches. It resides in the heart and has an upward motion which is sometimes called the ascending air (Udana Wayu). The navel is its central point of distribution throughout the whole body, functioning with the greatest strength at the tip of the nose, the head, navel, and great toes. This energy is consumed in the assimilation of food, in digestion, in the action of all vital organs, in the maintenance of the proper temperature of the body in the midst of excessive cold or heat. The taking of anything inside oneself is the work of Prana. It is by the power of Prana that one inhales, swallows, or even opens one's mouth. It is Prana which enables the eyes to see, the ears to hear, the nose to smell, the tongue to taste, the skin to feel. It is the motion of the Vital Air (Prana) in the Nadis (channels) that awakens consciousness—consciousness which is all-pervading but latent. Jiva (soul) is pure consciousness. The feeling-consciousness is the same, but more heavily veiled. The motive power in the world of thinking lies in the world of feeling. In Prana there is no intellect. Only feeling, or awareness, resides in Prana.

The mental phase of Prana is to take in and control. If, for one reason or another, Prana recedes from any part of the body, that part loses its power of action. This is called local death. It is thus that one becomes deaf, dumb, or blind, or has the digestive apparatus go wrong. Death is caused by the outgoing of Prana; the gasping of a dying man is known as the reversed breath. At death the exit of the Prana is by way of the eyes, ears, nose, navel, rectum, urethra, or fontanel. Its tendency is to leave the body at the point where the mind dwells or where the feelings reside. The air continually flows through the body, causing suffering. Therefore, the Yogi strives to stop this incessant flow of air.

The whole aim of the Swara Shastra is to expound the qualities and attributes of the Tattwas (Life Principles) and to inform the student in all their functions. As soon as one has succeeded in regulating the Breath, one will be able to understand all its parts and phases, which is the special art of Swarodaya, the Science of the Tattwas. Just as some Yogis spend their entire lives practising nothing but Hatha Yoga, there are some who devote their entire lives to the study and practice of the Swarodaya.

It will be found that one should combine both.

3

The breath in the right nostril is said to be hot, and that flowing in the left nostril is said to be cold. Therefore the right Nadi is called the Sun breath or Pingala, and the left Nadi is called the Moon breath or Ida. The energy which flows in the right nostril produces heat in the body. It is Katabolic, afferent, and accelatory to the organs of the body. The energy in the left nostril has a cooling effect ; it is anabolic, efferent, and inhibitory to the body organs. It increases nutrition and strength.

The breath alternates between the two nostrils. If this action is normal, the breath will alternate approximately every hour and fifty minutes. This normal action is the case only after one has perfected Pranayama. With the average person, all such changes of the breath vary a great deal, and are influenced by wrong habits, wrong diet, disease, and similar causes. Everything has some effect on the breath, diverting it from its normal flow. When the breath continues for a period longer than one hour and fifty minutes in one nostril, it is an indication of a derangement, due to an excess of heat or cold. This alternating breath is for the purpose of maintaining an equilibrium in the body temperature. Nasal breathing warms the air far more than mouth breathing by reason of the large area utilized in the breathing process.

Our body is a miniature counterpart of the whole Universe. The Sun and Moon, as they move always in their northern and southern orbits in the Macrocosm, are at the same time travelling in the Microcosm through Ida and Pingala during the day and night. The Moon, travelling in Ida, sprinkles its nectar of dew over the whole system ; while the Sun, travelling through Pingala, dries out the entire system. The meeting of the Sun and Moon at the Muladhara (lowest vital centre) is called Amabashya, the New Moon day. Close to this centre, the Kundalini (psychic energy) sleeps in Adharkunda. If anyone, with his mind under control, is able to confine the Moon in its place and the Sun in its place, so that the Moon is unable to shed its nectar, and the Sun is unable to dry it out, while the nectar of the body is dried from the fires of the Swadhisthana Chakra (the second centre of the body), the Kundalini will awaken by itself.

The alternation of the breath is affected by the mucous membrane in the head becoming hot and swollen on the side in which the air is not flowing. The membrane is in this condition at every change of breath from one nostril to the other. The followers of Swarodaya claim to be able to calculate the exact time of day and to determine the nature of events by the rhythmic erectility of the nasal mucous membrane, which is so clocklike in its regularity of becoming turgid in the functioning of a perfect body.

4

From twelve midnight until twelve noon, Prana flows in the nerves; because of this, the nervous energy is most active during this period. From twelve noon until midnight it flows in the blood vessels, which have a correspondingly greater strength during this period. At noon and midnight this energy becomes equal in both systems of Nadis. With sunset, Prana has passed into the blood vessels in full strength; at dawn, it passes into the spine, in accordance with the course of the sun (solar current of Prana).

In perfect health there is a balance of Prana in the Nadis. This means that the positive and negative currents flow in regular order and in definite channels. The operation of Free Will and certain other forces changes the nature of the local Prana, affecting the negative and positive flow in varying degrees. The character of this flow is the truest indication of a perfect record of the Tattwic changes in the body. Health is the result of this balance, and disease of the disruption of this balance. The Yogi makes an effort to bring these currents into order.

A breath of over twenty-four hours in one nostril warns a person that illness is near at hand. If it lasts over a longer period, it means that the illness will be a serious one. If one nostril should work continually for two or three days, the individual may count on a violent illness. This condition is caused by the fact that the ganglia of some particular nerve centre is being overworked as the result of the breath remaining in that particular centre for a longer period than is normal.

There are five important nerve centres in the body, starting from the base of the spine: Muladhara, Swadhis-thahna, Manipura, Anahata, and Vishuddha, all in the spinal cord. Everything must have a vehicle, and these Chakras (centres) are the vehicles of special kinds of consciousness. The characteristics of the energy and its function in each centre are classified thus: Prithivi (Earth), Apa (Water), Agni (Fire), Wayu (Air), Akasha (Ether). Though these are given here in their English rendering, they are far from being understood in the West. All five centres influence the breath, each affecting the flow according to the bodily habits and activities of the individual. In the normal state, at full development, these nerve currents cause the breath to flow 960 times an hour. On the other hand, when one nostril is completely closed, one knows immediately that the breath (nerve current) is in the Prithivi (earth centre) or Muladhara Chakra.

Each of these currents influences the element of the body according to the centre most active at the time. If Prana is circulating in Apa (water), the fluids of the body are being acted upon; the same holds good for the other centres. The exercises and practices of Yoga are used to liberate the movements of Prana in these centres, developing them in order to reveal the powers that lie hidden in them. Each Chakra (centre) has a given number of important Nadis which are called petals. Quite apart from their physical functions, they have a definite metaphysical aspect, of which the Yogi learns as he progresses with his practices.

5

In dreamless sleep, Prana sleeps in the blood vessels, in the pericardium, and in the hollow of the heart. Whenever Prana is agitated, or in motion, touching the Nadis, the ordinary state of consciousness is manifested. The regulated motion of Vital Air (Prana) will awaken greater consciousness, light, wisdom, and that latent power which pervades the entire body. The five Vital Airs originate in the active attributes of Akasha (Ether), while their elements—Prana, Apana, Samana, Udana, and Vyana—constitute what is designated as the Life Sack (Linga Sharira). In the Prana Gopala Tapani-Upanishad, it is asserted: " Air which is one becomes five on entering the world, and is so manifested in each body." In order to suspend the active phenomena of life for a single moment, it is necessary to have control over these energies.

The Yogi maintains a check on the breath at all times of special action, in order to make his every effort more effective. If he practises this continually, it will eventually become automatic.

It is always well to have a knowledge of the Tattwa that is flowing at any particular time ; its presence has considerable influence on the outcome of the particular action at the time. A knowledge of the nature of this action will often enable one to avoid or avert an illness, and help one to maintain a sound state of health.

There are several simple methods to be used in the beginning to change the flow of the breath. The Yogi will sometimes plug up the desired nostril with a piece of cotton. Another easy method is to place a little pressure under the arm-pit on the side of the particular nostril that you need to close. This may be accomplished by placing the arm-pit over a chair and pressing tightly against it. If this pressure is maintained for a few minutes, the breath will begin to flow in the opposite nostril. Yet another effective method is to manipulate the main nerve of the large toe at the ankle of the foot

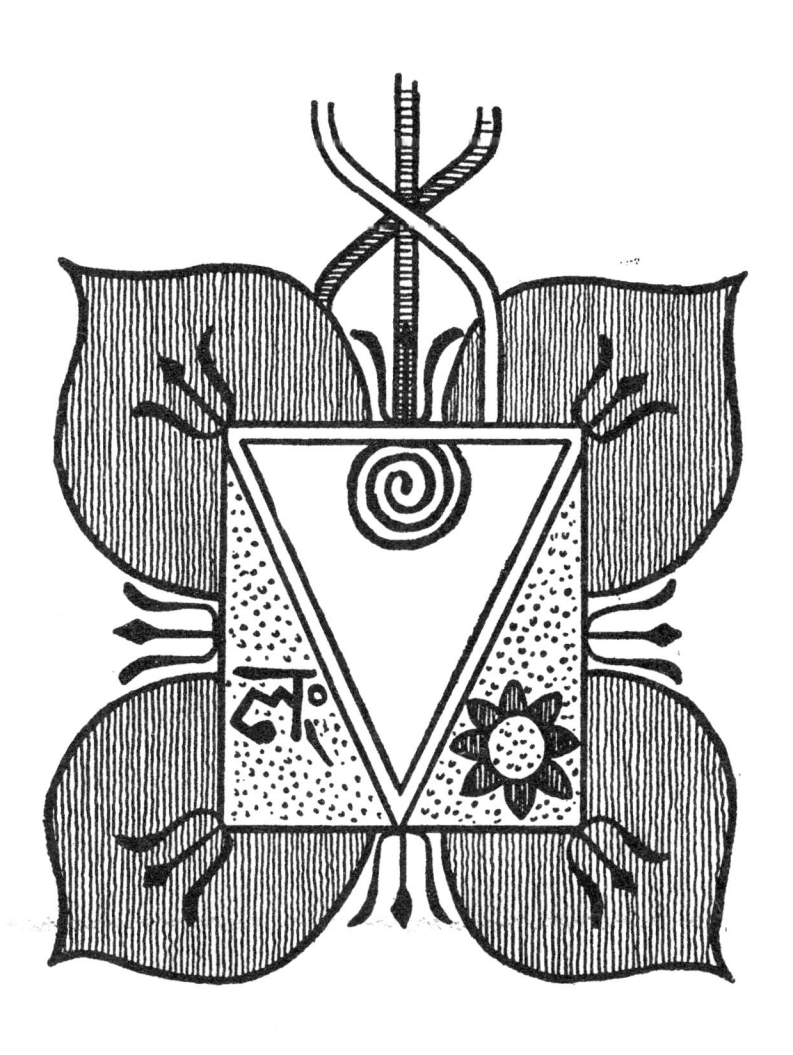

MULADHARA CHAKRA

on the side on which you want the breath to flow. Another simple method is to sit on the floor and draw up the knee to a position where it is possible to place it within the arm-pit; then, by leaning on it, the breath will begin to flow in the opposite nostril. Or you may sit down on the floor and press your shoulder against the wall, or put pressure on the nerve under the calf of the leg. Frequently, Yogis carry a short crutch with them, upon which they can lean while seated; thus, they can keep the breath flowing in a specific nostril at all times.

By continual practice, it is possible to change the breath very quickly. In most instances, ten minutes will be found sufficient. The Yogi instructs one to make it a rule to sleep on the left side, so that the food lying in the bag of the stomach on the affected side may be thoroughly digested before it passes into the intestines. This is assured him by the fact that it also keeps the Pingala (Sun Breath) flowing, aiding the digestive fires. For the acquisition of psychic powers, the Yogi places great confidence in the Sun Breath.

6

We had kept up a continuous conversation from tea-time till midnight, without once having moved from our positions. Then we had a good-night cup of tea. I had still two hours ahead of me for noting in my diary the substance of our discussion; it was a daily habit to which I strictly adhered.

They did not approve of any method which called for immediate transcription of things said and heard. Their students were expected to memorize word for word from oral instruction. It is possible for the native student to memorize literally volumes of spoken words. Indeed, this is the manner in which their teachings have come down to us through the centuries. There are written records, to be sure; but these suffer from modern interpretation. New meanings, having no relation to the old, are given them. And when, as it often

More About the Science of Breath

happens, the text has been rewritten several times, the whole original significance is gone.

The instruction I received resulted from my asking questions. At the very beginning I had been told that there was no such thing as a " silly question " ; I was taught that the asking of questions was regarded as a real indication of my growth. It was important to frame the question in the proper way ; it was a sort of key to one's intelligence and sincerity. There was no particular system in this question-and-answer method, but there was a realism about it that was very effective in learning the essentials. My newly acquired knowledge became an integral part of me in a manner that would have been impossible with any other method. The recording of what was said in the course of the day had its use for me, however ; for it helped to a fuller comprehension of the teachings imparted me.

Before parting with my host that night, it had been decided that I should remain with him for the rest of the week, after which we would journey together to visit the Swamaji, who had gone to the jungle hermitage of his teacher. Perhaps, there, I could begin my practical work as a disciple of Yoga. I bade my friend good night in the customary way of folding the hands together and bowing slightly.

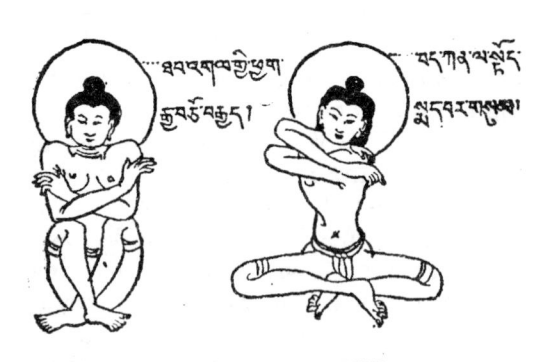

CHAPTER XII

IMPORTANCE OF PRANAYAMA

I

THOUGH I sat up very late the night before, I did not forego my early morning silence. There was a standing order to have my tea brought at five.

On my stroll that morning I reflected on what was happening to me. I was trying to peer through the illusion of reality, trying to get a glimpse of the law of Karma that was functioning; for it was quite apparent to me that all my activities were the result of the fulfilment of some law. It was not for me to decide what I should do. It was for me to fulfil the destiny which guided my steps.

I was aware that before long I should have to take up the strenuous discipline of the life of a Yogi. Would I be able to stand the strain? I was ambitious, determined, and I felt conscious of a dynamic energy. Nevertheless, I was also conscious of the warning the American doctors had given me immediately after my illness. Here was I, weighing the balance of knowledge between the East and the West. The Eastern teachings gave me the assurance that there was no danger; deep within me I felt that they were right, a judgment so far confirmed by my triumphs. Yet the word of Death came echoing to me from the West, ever cautioning me to beware.

My mind was becoming crowded with more and more

Importance of Pranayama

information; I was becoming increasingly aware that it might lead me away from the Truth. The very energy and time consumed were taking me farther and farther from my goal; for all that is purely mental is an illusion. It is true that the only way to pour sense knowledge into the inner consciousness is through the mind; that is its divine function. It is the instrument of precision through which one gains entry to the Inner Self. But one is constantly being lost in the mind itself. This was my danger. My awareness of this, however, acted as a safeguard against my being caught in the fatal snare of Maya (illusion).

2

The day before our departure, my Tantrik friend spent an entire morning in imparting to me his ideas on Pranayama. He tried to give me a very simple, clear picture of the Tantrik teachings appertaining to this science. Much of it I had read or heard before. The chief value of his talk, however, was that it presented an excellent review, clearing up in particular those aspects which were still vague in my mind.

Prana means breath, Yama means pause; hence, Pranayama is simply a properly regulated form of an otherwise irregular and hurried flow of air. It controls the triple process of inhalation (Puraka), suspension (Kumbhaka), and exhalation (Rechaka). It is the practice of inhaling to one's capacity, suspending as long as possible, and then exhaling until the lungs are as empty as possible.

Pranayama is one of the most important practices of all forms of Yoga; it is a process by which one can isolate the Inner Self from the influx and influence of worldly thoughts. It is a sort of tool for reaching the finer forces that function in the body. Its aim is to enable the Yogi to obtain control over the nervous system; it is this control that gradually enables him to dominate the Prana, or Vital energy, and the mind. This is the real object of the practice, which is a vehicle for the revelation of aspects of life and nature which cannot be had in any other way.

The body must co-operate in the work of the Yogi. There is a saying that " He who fasts and he who eats too much, he who does not sleep and he who sleeps too much, he who works too much and he who does not work—none of these can be an adept." A Sadhaka (one who practises) needs solitude. This is essential. For the practice of Pranayama and mind culture, one must have a place of retirement, where, if possible, one can be alone with nature, unconditioned by the refinements of this day and age. The most desirable retreat is a small chamber of about six feet square, free from ornamentation and shut off from noise. If this is unavailable, the next best thing is a quiet room, a cellar, an attic, or a retreat in the woods or in a canyon. It should have good air, be neither too cold nor too hot, and it should be close to one's source of food. The ideal quarters would be a cave some six feet square, near a sparkling pool of water. It is in such a place that the higher forms of Yoga training are undertaken. To be sure, an ideal place for the practice of Yoga can hardly be expected to-day, so it is necessary to select the most advantageous available and make the most of it.

My Trantrik friend pointed out that perhaps the only place left in the world where it would be possible for one to go and find the ideal place for meditation would be Tibet. But Tibet is beyond the hope of almost all of us. As is well known, they do not permit foreigners to enter the country, except in very rare instances. Consequently one should make the most of what there is available for him, and let Time solve his future problems.

The place finally resolved upon should not be too far removed from such necessities as food, water, etc., and it must be a spot protected from curious and troublesome people. It is better to live a lonely life than to have the campanionship of the stupid and worldly-minded ; even one's own family should be seen as rarely as possible.

Importance of Pranayama

Strength is the only important limitation in any Yoga practice. Physical capacity alone limits the frequency, but one should measure his own limitations carefully, not attempting too much, but holding to the amount chosen at each practice until it becomes easy, then increase by small stages.

Yoga should be practised only when the mind and body are fresh and when untroubled by evil or carnal thoughts. Chastity is essential for storing vital energy and in the case of a married man his wife can be most helpful if she is sympathetic and understanding. But in no circumstances must the practice of Yoga limit the wife's happiness, to which she has a right. One must strive to "be in the world but not of it," always grave but joyful, never jealous nor vain. But if evil thoughts enter the mind, do not use will power to drive them away; simply ignore them. By remaining indifferent and passive they will gradually leave as mysteriously as they came. But at such time no Yoga should be practised; it is best to indulge in some form of physical exercise. There need be no cause for anxiety, however, as these are obstacles met and conquered by all Yogis.

The preparation of the body may begin at any season of the year, but one should begin the practice of Pranayama in the spring or fall. In winter and summer diseases are more frequent, but in the spring and fall the air is pure and one is not so likely to derange his vital principles. Changes in the air greatly affect the functions of the human body and have a corresponding effect on the mind. The body is most vigorous, active, and strong and the spirit most brisk and lively when the sky is serene and unclouded and the wind east, north-east, or south-east. Just so is warm dry air superior to cold moist conditions. Intense cold obstructs the fine vessels of the head, lungs, and joints. A morbid condition is often the result of continued humidity.

3

A sound body is the foundation of a sound mind. The purification of the Nadis (nerves) is the first step. Pranayama is of great assistance in this. The cleansing of the Nadis may be accomplished by Pranayama in three months, and if the person happens to be in good physical condition at the start, it can be done in even less time.

Without purified Nadis there can be no accomplishment in Pranayama. One may practise twice a day—morning and evening; or three times a day—morning, noon, and evening; or four times a day—morning, noon, evening, and midnight; or eight times in the twenty-four hours by practising every three hours. At a minimum, it should be practised over a period of forty-eight minutes twice daily, and extended as soon as possible to four times in twenty-four hours.

All practice should be done at a time when one is neither hungry nor satiated with food. One should avoid practice when tired.

Again and again it must be stressed that the accomplishment of Yoga is defeated by over-eating, over-exertion, indulgence in a morning cold bath, eating at night, limiting one's diet to fruit, excessive company, irregularity of habits, etc. Excessive application brings distraction, immoderate sleep induces sluggishness, dulls the mind, obstructs the memory, and causes the disintegration of the physical and spiritual powers of man.

Sleep in the daytime deranges the three Doshas (bodily principles of Wayu, Pitta, Kapha (nervous energy, heat of metabolism, and lymphatic function); so it should be strictly avoided.

The student should rise every morning at the peep of dawn, or about four a.m. Rising early in the morning is not at all difficult, once the habit has been formed; indeed, it comes just as natural as rising at nine. He is to begin his practice by doing some Asanas (postures). Sarvangasana (a posture) should be done last, so that

Importance of Pranayama

Jalandhara (chin lock) may be accomplished more easily. Mirtasana (corpse pose) may be done whenever one is fatigued. One should sit in the same place at the same time each day, keep the eyes closed, hold the body and head erect.

Regularity is absolutely essential. At the minimum, one should set a course of three months' practice. Within that period a very good control may be attained.

The practice of Pranayama up to four periods a day is advisable as soon as the student is capable. This standard should be maintained for three months. The ideal standard of practice is that of four times during the twenty-four hours: 4 a.m. to 6 a.m., 10 a.m. to 12 m., 4 p.m. to 6 p.m., and 10 p.m. to 12 p.m. This should be continued until it is possible for one to do eighty rounds of Kumbhaka at each sitting. This will make 320 rounds over the period of twenty-four hours. The student should start with ten on the first day, increasing the practice at the rate of four rounds a day. In three months he should be able to reach the maximum. Vaschaspti, a renowned authority on Yoga, gives thirty-six counts (seconds) as the lowest ratio for Pranayama. This he designates as mild. Seventy-two seconds he looks upon as moderate, and 108 as intense Pranayama. For the tender initiate twelve counts are considered inferior, twenty-four middling, and thirty-six superior.

He who has a knowledge of Breath in his mind has a fortune at his feet, for Breath determines the pressure behind all activity and circulation. It is one of the two causes of the activity of the mind, the other being desire. Through the regulation of breath, Karma acquired in this life, as well as that acquired in past lives, can be burnt up. From experience it will be learned that Pranayama destroys all sin and the world of illusion in the same manner that a fire consumes dry wood. The fire which is latent in wood ignites only with friction, and so the wisdom that is latent in all living souls arises only by the practice of Pranayama. By Pranayama the power of levitation can be acquired, diseases cured, spiritual energy awakened. Calmness and mental powers are obtained. The Path for one who practises Pranayama is filled with bliss.

When one finally acquires complete control over the sympathetic nervous system, one becomes master of his body and can die at will. One is certain to meet Brahma (the Overself) by the continuous practice of Pranayama for a year. Without it no Yogi can realize the illumination of his soul during the Kali Yuga.

The object of these breathing exercises is, first, to control the local Prana-Wayu and to stop organic action. All the forces arising from the inside must be controlled in order that the mind may become "one-pointed" toward the Supreme Consciousness. Later the entire involuntary system is made voluntary. The climax is Samadhi, when there is complete suspension of animation.

By Kumbhaka the efferent fibres of the Vagus are stimulated, resulting in the stimulation of the Vagal Centre in the Medulla Oblongata, which results in a slowing down of the heart's action. If this is carried far enough it is believed that one can stop the entire action of the heart. This nerve has a more extensive distribution than any other Cranal nerve. It contains more sensory and motor fibres. It supplies the organs of the voice and of respiration with both motor and sensory fibres, and it supplies the pharynx, œsophagus, heart, and stomach with motor fibres. The stimulation of this nerve at its centre in the Medulla Oblongata causes inhibitions of such organs as the heart, lungs, and larynx and the acceleration of the movements of the stomach. This vagal centre is also excited by the stimulation of its afferent fibres, of the nasal mucous membrane, larynx, and lungs. Kundalini Shakti (nervous energy) may be excited when the Vagus nerve is violently vibrated by Pranayama.

When one inhales, he is taking in Prana. The more Prana one can take in the more vitality he will possess. In the practice of Pranayama it is important to

Importance of Pranayama

observe consciously everything which takes place in the phenomena of breathing. Another important principle is to create always a certain amount of "Pranic" pressure in the system. This is done by inhaling during a given period a greater amount of air than normally. The ratio between the period of inhalation and the lasting effect of "pressure" is one to sixty. Thus a person who takes long, deep, and heavy breaths for one minute will create a pressure for one hour. That is to say, the value of the deep breathing will not be exhausted for approximately one hour. For a period of twenty-four hours one must practise for a period of twenty-four minutes. Some people find it impossible to practise for twenty-four minutes at a time and so cut the time in half, practising twice daily. The Yogi who is capable of reducing the normal length of the exhalation will enjoy perfect health and acquire spiritual powers.

4

It is due to the working of a necessary law of life that the mind undergoes the various changes in waking and sleeping states. With the approach of darkness the ordinary physical mood is altered and the positive forces in Nature are gathered up. This results in a lessening of sense activity, they no longer receiving impressions from without and a sleep creeps over them. The average amount of "absolute rest" during a night's sleep is claimed to be only eleven and one-half minutes. The remainder of the time spent in so-called sleep, the individual is subject to muscular and mental action. Sleep, as a rule, has an overpowering influence on the mind by reason of its Tamaguna quality.

In Yoga it is taught that wakefulness, dreaming, and dreamless sleep are the result of a certain degree of temperature at which sensuous organs ordinarily work, all being under cardiac temperature. In Sanskrit the phenomenon is called Sadhaka Titta. When the negative Ida (cold nerve current) has reached its limit, that is, has become predominant over Pingala (hot nerve current), consciousness sleeps in the heart. When the positive current Pingala reaches its daily extreme, the action of the sense organs is no longer synchronized with the several internal modifications of the Tattwas and then we have the manifestation of wakefulness in all its activity. Nature is ever seeking to maintain a balance in these two elements of hot and cold. When the Yogi, through the power of Prana or Mantra, makes active this cardiac temperature he is able to achieve such results as his competency permits.

The Buddhists teach that too much sleep destroys all religious merit, and they claim that anyone will find an occasional vigil very helpful.

From the perfection of Pranayama follows a decrease of sleep, and the Yogi finds his solid body as volatile as air. He never perspires, his semen dries up, and the seminal force ascends to return as nectar (Amriti of Shiva, Shakti). He becomes free of disease and sorrow. There is neither increase nor decrease in the Vital Principles. When this last stage arrives the Yogi may with impunity be irregular in his diet and his other habits without any injurious results following his deviation from the former rigid rules. He may "eat, drink, and be merry" without any evil consequences.

By Pranayama one is able to live without air, food, or drink, and gain the power of levitation. The mind becomes calm and full of bliss. There is an exaltation of mental powers, and the spiritual energy is awakened. With the control of Prana, Agni (bodily heat) in the body will increase daily. With the increase of Agni, food will be easily digested. With food properly digested, Rasa (metamorphosed food essence) increases. With the increase of Rasa, Dhatus (bodily root principles) increase, and with the increase of Dhatus, Wisdom increases. The sins during scores of years are burned up.

What is known as total suspension requires thirteen and one-half minutes. This is Samadhi. It is said that

Importance of Pranayama

the senses become suspended when one can perform Kumbhaka for a period of ten minutes and forty-eight seconds. Gradually the Yogi will be able to suspend his breath for one and one-half hours, when he will attain all of his longed-for powers. In fact, there is nothing in the world which does not become possible for him.

The Yogi can now enjoy the wonderful state of Pratyahara, when he suspends his breath for three hours.

5

Lunch had come and gone without my having any realization of the passage of time, so intent was I upon the teachings. It was now time to rest until the cool of the afternoon. It was still very warm, even though it was fall. The heat at midday was as great as that of New York or Chicago at the same hour of mid-July. In India this is considered comfortable, and I found it so. At teatime we would continue the discussion on Pranayama. At that time my Tantrik friend was going to relate the more important techniques used in accomplishing the art of Pranayama.

It is scarcely necessary to say that throughout the morning I had been living virtually in another world. It was my constant dream that it might come to pass that I should taste of the illumination of the heart of which he had spoken. I felt certain that if I were permitted to follow the discipline I could attain the initial state of inner peace, resulting in joy and bliss forever after.

Could I hold to the discipline? My opportunity was approaching.

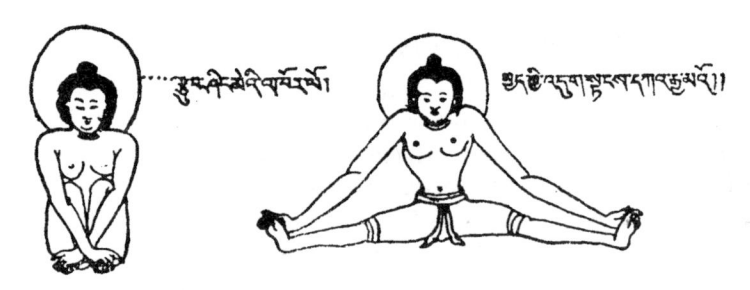

CHAPTER XIII

EXERCISES TO CURE DISEASES AND TO EXTEND YOUTH

I

In the afternoon the first practice taken up was Kapalabhati, which is, as my teacher explained, not a Pranayama in the strictest sense, but an essential exercise which must be used. It is a process of washing and purifying the nerves and cleansing the body of Kapha (phlegm). It is one of the six processes of cleansing the Nadis and a practice which also holds considerable spiritual value. There is no regular Kumbhaka in this practice. The Lotus Pose (Padmasana) is assumed. The exercise consists only of Rechaka and Puraka. Rechaka (exhalation) is the principal part of the exercise, while Puraka (inhalation) is only supplementary.

A vigorous practice of Kapalabhati for a few minutes will vibrate every tissue of the body. This will become more and more violent as the exercise is pushed farther with its original vigour until it becomes difficult to control one's posture. This is why it is so necessary to do the practice in the Lotus Pose which has the foot lock. It would be impossible otherwise to hold one's seat throughout the practice. The spine should be held erect and the hands rested on the knees. In Kapalabhati there is a play of the abdominal muscles and diaphragm. These are suddenly and vigorously contracted, giving an inward push to the abdominal viscera. The diaphragm then recedes into the thoracic cavity which expels all the air from the lungs.

In normal respiration inhalation is active while the process of exhalation is passive. In Kapalabhati this is reversed. Rechaka and Puraka are performed in quick succession by a sudden and vigorous instroke of the abdominal muscles. This is instantly followed by a relaxation of these muscles. Rechaka occupies about one fourth of the time of Puraka. The relaxation is a passive act, while the contraction is a very active one. No time is allowed between these acts until a round is completed. In the beginning a round should have ten expulsions. Generally three rounds are performed at each sitting, a sitting being performed twice each day, morning and evening. As a rule ten expulsions may be added each week until 120 expulsions can be done at each round.

Between successive rounds normal respiration is allowed to afford the needed rest. Those who feel themselves fit are permitted to double the usual number, but the minimum should be three rounds of three minutes each at a sitting. Under no condition should a strain be placed on the system. It is imperative to remember this.

One should pay attention only to his abdominal muscles, the mind being centred on the administering of the abdominal strokes against the centre of the abdomen at the navel where Spiritual Energy is stored (Kundalini). This concentration must be maintained throughout the practice. Eventually the nervous system will become spiritually active. This will be manifest by a throbbing sensation and a form of a serene light will glow at this particular centre, seen of course only with the mind's eye.

Great quantities of carbon dioxide gas are eliminated and similar quantities of oxygen are absorbed into the system, making the blood much richer and renewing the tissues of the body. Kapalabhati has no parallel as an exercise of great oxygen value. It corrects all ailments which arise from cold and is extremely helpful in arresting the approach of old age. Its nerve culture is very efficacious and its effect on the circulation and metabolism is of considerable importance.

As well as being a nerve-cleansing process, it is also practised for awakening certain nerve centres which make the practice of Pranayama more efficient by quieting the respiratory centre. A few rounds of this practice should be performed daily before doing Pranayama. Five minutes is sufficient to induce a state of trance when one has fully developed the art of Kapalabhati.

The speed depends on one's practice, and thoroughness should never be sacrificed for speed. Starting with one expulsion a second, it may be developed into two a second, which is a good rate for a normal person. It is possible to develop it to a point when one can do 200 a minute, but to exceed this renders the expirations so shallow that all efficiency is lost. The vigour of the expulsions must be constantly watched and never reduced for the sake of speed. Vigour, speed, measuring of a single round, the number to a sitting, the total amount done in a day, should be judiciously determined according to the capacity of each individual.

I will just mention two other methods frequently used to cleanse the Nadis. One, which takes a few months, is accomplished by holding the right nostril and drawing in the breath hard through the left nostril, then suspending as long as one can comfortably, exhaling as slowly as possible through the right nostril. Repeat, reversing the process by inhaling through the right nostril. Practise this four times a day, morning, noon, sundown, midnight, six or eight times at each sitting. This practice makes the body light, increasing the appetite, producing secret sounds in the head. When this occurs the student should stop. The second method is to pucker the lips, pushing them out a little, then inhale slowly through the mouth and try to feel the air contacting the back part of the throat. When the inhalation is completed, swallow, then suspend with the pressure low in the abdomen. This second practice cures indigestion as well as other bodily diseases, thereby contributing to one's longevity.

Breathing hard induces the Apas (water) and Prithivi (earth) Tattwas. By tying the right arm above the elbow and the right leg below the knee it is possible to excite these Tattwas, and especially that of Prithivi.

2

Suryabheda Kumbhaka (Secret of the Sun) was the next process my Tantrik friend explained to me that afternoon.

There are four Bhedas: Surya, Ujjayi, Sitali, and Bhastrika. Suryabheda increases the heat of the body. By this process the Yogi cures diseases which depend on an insufficiency of oxygen. The practice rids one of pulmonary, cardiac, and dropsical diseases. It cleanses the frontal sinuses, destroys disorders of Wayu, awakens Kundalini, and prevents bodily decay and premature death.

The technique is simple. It is a process of breathing in through the right nostril. After inhaling to full capacity, swallow, suspend, and do the chin lock (Jalandhara). Hold the Kumbhaka as long as possible, but do not strain. Then with a slow unbroken force exhale the breath through the left nostril. Repeat. It is important to keep some control and tension on the abdominal muscles. By the practice of putting pressure in the solar-plexus the mental side is developed. By putting pressure in any part of the trunk breathing is regulated and Kapha (phlegm) evaporated. This practice may be started with ten Pranayamas a day, increasing it five daily to a maximum of eighty. When the student has fully developed it, he may continue repeating it even more so long as perspiration does not burst forth from the roots of the hair and the finger tips, while maintaining the Kumbhaka. Perspiration is a healthy sign and preserves the body from disease as well as removing them.

Padmasana or Siddhasana may be used for this practice. After practising Suryabhedana one should do Ujjayi, Sitkari, Sitali, and finally Bhastrika. It matters but little whether or not one does other practices.

Ujjayi means "pronounced loudly." Start this practice by complete exhalation through the mouth. Then begin. Ujjayi is a deep-chest breathing exercise: take in deep breaths with the glottis slightly closed, then suspension, followed by a slow exhalation until rhythmic breathing starts. This practice increases the heat of the body. Any posture is suitable. The breath is to be drawn in through both nostrils, expanding the chest, and partially closing the glottis, making a sobbing sound of a low but sweet and uniform pitch. The abdominal muscles should be kept under control by slight contraction, which is maintained throughout the inhalation.

On completion of the inhalation, which must be smooth and uniform, a swallowing action is executed. Kumbhaka and Jalandhara follow. The real advantage lies in the Kumbhaka, but this should not be stressed to the point of suffocation nor to the point where it becomes impossible to control a smooth well-regulated exhalation, through the left nostril, or through both nostrils, with the glottis partially closed, making the same sound as before.

The period of exhalation should take twice the time of inhalation and one should seek to prolong the duration at each round. In the beginning about four rounds a minute is a suitable pace. At the end of the practice period one should not be overly tired. The breath which fills the mouth should be swallowed and taken to the region of the solar plexis where a sort of belching act is accomplished without opening the nostrils or the mouth. Let the air rise again and go down again. It will aid in awakening all the Nadis from the throat to the navel. This practice is of great help when Kundalini begins to move and endeavours to move up.

To prepare for the practice, a week or so may be given to Ujjayi, leaving off the Kumbhaka. Seven rounds are sufficient at the beginning, adding three

Exercises to Cure Diseases and Extend Youth

rounds each week or more or less according to capacity. The maximum number of daily rounds should be 320, distributed over two to four sittings. Two hundred and forty are sufficient for one interested solely in the physical aspects of the practice. Its perfection will protect one from diseases, such as: indigestion, dysentery, consumption, cough, fever, enlarged spleen, and nervous diseases.

Sitkari is the process of breathing only through the mouth, which has the effect of keeping the body cool. It is done by drawing the air through the mouth, making all the noise possible, then immediately exhaling. It is important to keep the teeth firmly pressed together, suspending the tongue so that it does not touch the palate, the bottom of the mouth or the teeth. On inhaling the pull should be from the lower abdomen to full capacity of the lungs. This is to be done fifty to eighty times and best practised at night. Take a glass of warm milk about twenty minutes before beginning. This practice oxygenates the blood, cures insomnia removes hunger and thirst, indolence, and sleep, and generally contributes to the comfort of the system. It increases the beauty and vigour of the body and cures phthisis. By breathing this moist air the body soon becomes free of all diseases. It is by this Kumbhaka that a Yogi enables himself to become cold-blooded and independent in being. In six months, it is said, one can acquire poetic genius, having perfected this exercise. A Yogi perfected in all other respects also attains clairvoyance and clairaudience.

Sitali Kumbhaka is a process of Pranayama accomplished by inhaling through the mouth and exhaling through the nostrils. This also keeps the body cool. It is equivalent to Sitkari with Kumbhaka added. Either method may be used without a Kumbhaka when it is desired to add only moisture to the system

After turning the tongue back with its tip on the soft palate, inspire by the combined exertion of the tongue and the soft palate This is called Manduka Mudra

(Frog Mudra), because it is after the manner of a frog. After inhaling, suspend the breath before exhaling through both nostrils while relaxing the whole system. This form of Kumbhaka is in imitation of the snake. It is necessary to live on milk, Ghee and cold water. It will promote a love of study and retirement and bring about the power of self-trance.

If Pranayama has previously been perfected, one month's practice will give sufficient power to repair the effects of injury, add tenacity to life, and free the body from the dangers of fevers. It is by the practice of Sitali Kumbhaka that snakes shed their skins and by the practice of Bhastrika snakes produce their hissing noise. Splenitis and several organic diseases can be cured by this practice. One will be able to endure the deprivation of air, water, and food. He will be endowed with the ability to renew his skin, enhancing his beauty. It will make him cold-blooded and it will be easy for him to spend his time in solitude and devotion.

A Yogi who can combine Apana with Prana is indeed happy, and if he can breathe pure air by fixing his tongue to his palate, he frees himself from ALL diseases. By drinking this water-saturated air daily, he becomes free from fatigue. When the Yogi has perfected his technique of Pranayama, if he practises for only a short time daily, there is no doubt he can free himself from diseases, old age, and attain a very long life.

When the Yogi can fill his entire intestinal canal with air, he acquires the power of fasting off his skin and altering his specific gravity at will. He can become plump or lean at will. He can become light or heavy at will.

Another method of performing this practice is to roll the tongue lengthwise, allowing it to protrude a little beyond the lips. The air is then drawn in very slowly, the lungs filled as far as is possible. Follow with the customary swallowing act before doing a Kumbhaka for a short time. The exhalation should be through both nostrils. One should mentally visualize the fact that the air goes to the mouth of Kundalini.

This method frees one from indigestion, colic, enlarged spleen, fevers, disorders of the bile, phlegm. It cures lung trouble, counteracts poisons, hunger and thirst, and fills one with a peculiar feeling of bliss. This Mudra is called Kaki Mudra (Crow Bill Mudra) and it should be practised at dawn and twilight. One will acquire an intuitive knowledge of the minds of others, an insight into the nature of objects and a knowledge of the deeper stream of life.

Bhastrika Kumbhaka preserves an even temperature of the body. This is equivalent to the practice of Kapalabhati with a Kumbhaka added. It is best to practise it in Padmasana; in the earlier stages, however, Siddhasana or Vajrasana may be used. In the final perfection of the practice it is absolutely essential to use Padmasana in order to be able to retain one's seat. After the correct posture, straighten the back and neck, inhale slowly until the stomach is fully expanded, then exhale forcibly through the nostrils. Then inhale and exhale rapidly with emphasis on the exhalation. Make a noise which can be felt in the throat, chest, and head. This is to be done twenty times or so, or until one is fatigued. Then inhale through the right nostril, filling the abdomen, suspend, and fix the gaze upon the tip of the nose. Kumbhaka is to be done just as long as one can do it comfortably. After the suspension, exhale through the left nostril and then inhale through the same nostril, again suspending the breath, and exhale through the right nostril. This completes one round.

Each expulsion of breath must be sudden. The automatic inhalation is much slower. The process imitates the action of a blacksmith's bellows. Practise slowly at the start, then gradually increase the number of Rechakas (exhalations), until there are 120 a minute. It is advisable to begin with only ten rounds, increasing according to individual capacity.

With each breath and heartbeat, the brain cerebrates. It increases in volume with each exhalation and decreases with each inhalation, which means, of course, that the brain is constantly rising and falling in volume. This motion is closely connected with the rapidity of blood circulation in the brain, giving a fresh and generous supply of blood to it. What takes place in the brain must of necessity take place in the other organs with the same modification. Respiration exerts a modification upon the circulation of the blood in the venous trunks. The vein in the neck will be suddenly emptied when the chest dilates to inspire. On the other hand, it will be seen to swell when the chest contracts. The more marked the respiratory movements, the more striking will be these movements.

When the Auricle contracts, the blood is driven to the head and when it dilates it is sent to the heart. As the motions of the Auricle are much more frequent than those of the Thorax, the beating of the jugular vein is very irregular. This is particularly the case during disease.

The increased blood circulation all over the body from the practice of Bhastrika tones up the entire nervous system. A prolonged practice arouses every atom of the body, setting the entire system in motion until it is wholly reconstructed and purified. In time, occult forces are awakened and one becomes a new and infinitely more powerful being.

In the beginning the bodily heat is increased by the quickened circulation, which is followed by a reduced bodily temperature due to profuse perspiration and the rapid and violent respiratory movements which end in Kumbhaka. When a lively circulation of the blood is accompanied by a free perspiration, impure matter is eliminated and the strength and nourishment of the body are better maintained. This will enable the mind and body to perform their functions with greater facility.

The practice should be done at least twice a day until a good heat is worked up or pressure is felt in the temples. Then one should rest before continuing. If fatigue is experienced during practice, fill the lungs through the right nostril, suspend as long as possible, and exhale through the left nostril.

This practice corrects any imbalance of Wayu, Pitta, or Kapha. It facilitates digestion, enriches the blood, and improves the action of the heart. A strong resistance to contagion and infectious diseases is built up. It is splendid for preventing fever, if one must live in swampy places or fever-infested districts. When it is done in preparation for such conditions, its effects will last for many months.

Bhastrika Kumbhaka enables the Yogi to alter his specific gravity at will. It increases his appetite, cures pulmonary and hepatic diseases, purifies the system, destroys the impurities which accumulate at the entrance of the Brahma Nadi, quickly awakens Kundalini, and affords him great pleasure. If it is practised ten or twenty times and each time followed by a Kumbhaka, it becomes an effective treatment for impotency. It is effective in so many ways because it gives a sort of electric shock to the whole system.

It is the finest exercise for the vascular and nervous systems that human genius has ever discovered. It awakens and electrifies the nervous system to an unimaginable extent. The rapid blood circulation in Bhastrika and the vibrations of the tissues of the entire body lead to a massage of nearly the whole of the nervous, muscular, and circulatory systems. To open the three superior valves of the Shakti Nadi, it is necessary to practise Bhastrika Kumbhaka.

Bhastrika performed plentifully breaks the three knots: the one in the pelvis which is called Brahma Granthi (situated in the Muladhara Chakra), the one at the navel which is known as Vishnu Granthi (situated in the Manipura Chakra), and the one between the eyes which is Rudra Granthi (situated in the Ajna Chakra). ALL of them are made to function freely by strenuous effort.

As soon as Kundalini has been moved, Bhastrika should be practised plentifully in order to awaken it.

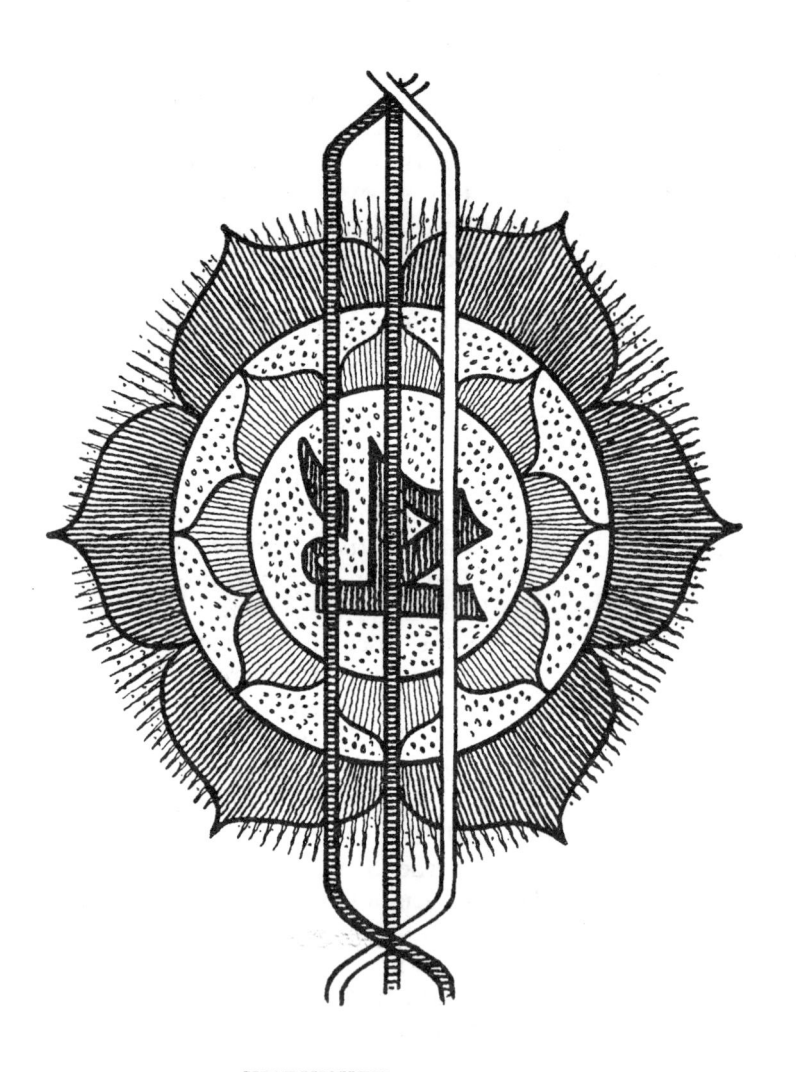

SVADHISHTHANA CHAKRA

When this has been perfected one may suit his own desire as to whether or no other Kumbhakas are practised. Bhastrika and Ujjayi are considered the best varieties of Pranayama. They should always follow after complete evacuation and a complete bath. It is advisable to use Ghee sparingly when practising Bhastrika. Buttermilk is permitted. The main meal should be in the middle of the day.

Suryabedha and Ujjayi produce heat. Sitkari and Sitali are cooling. Bhastrika preserves the normal temperature. Suryabedha destroys Wayu. Ujjayi destroys excess Kapha. Sitkari and Sitali destroy excess Pitta. Bhastrika makes for a balance of all three. Sitkari and Sitali are more useful in hot weather. Bhastrika may be done in all seasons.

Sahita Kumbhaka is of two sorts and is practised with or without Mantras. One takes his seat in Padmasana and closes the nostrils, the right one with the thumb, the left one with the little and ring fingers. It must never be done with the middle or index fingers. Now release the two fingers and inhale slowly, just as slowly as possible through the left nostril. When the lungs are filled, swallow the breath. This packs the air and gives the muscles of the throat a better tension to hold the inspired air. Then do the chin lock (Jalandhara) and suspend. The air is now held in the lungs just so long as one can without pain or suffocation, then it is slowly exhaled through the right nostril, while the left is kept closed with the two fingers. This is immediately followed by drawing the air in through the right nostril, retaining it and exhaling through the left, in the same manner as before. This alternation of inhaling and exhaling continues, finishing by exhaling through the left nostril. While practising, the mind is placed on the Fire Centre at the navel or upon the Nectar flowing from the Moon in the head or, if preferred, upon the flow of the breath through the nostrils.

This mode of Kumbhaka should be practised at the four quarters of the day. The Nadis and nervous system will become thoroughly purified if it is continued daily for three months. Once all the Nadis are purified, one will be free from all functional disorders, and will have stepped forth on the first stage in the practice of Yoga. His body will become harmoniously developed and emit a sweet scent, his appearance will be pleasing and handsome, he will be perpetually cheerful, have great courage, intense enthusiasm. His body will be handsome and full of strength and power. The practice should be continued until these signs make their appearance.

The ratio of the three breaths should be one second inhalation to four seconds suspension and two seconds exhalation. According to the student's capacity the practice can last to forty-eight minutes for each of four periods daily, always ending by exhaling through the left nostril, which establishes equipoise. At first it is advisable to practise only Puraka and Rechaka without Kumbhaka. After about a week one may introduce a Kumbhaka, but there should never be any haste. Puraka, Kumbhaka and Rechaka must be adjusted to individual capacity with great caution. Experience and constant practice alone can assure success. A systematic routine is positively essential. This will guarantee immediate increase in one's Kumbhaka. This discipline must be followed in the practice of Asana (posture), Japa (recitation of Mantras), concentration, mediation, and all the other practices of Yoga. Puraka (inhalation) causes growth and nourishment and equalizes the vital principles. Kumbhaka (retention) causes stability and increases the security of life ; and Rechaka (exhalation) removes all sin and gives complete control over the body.

One should always come out of the practice invigorated and fully refreshed. It must never be carried to the point of fatigue. There must always be exhilaration of the Spirit. The body must not be exposed to draught, and it is advisable not to take a bath immediately following the practice. A complete rest for thirty minutes is usual. The best results will be obtained if

Exercises to Cure Diseases and Extend Youth 167

one particular form of practice is selected and developed to the highest possible degree before trying to do them all.

Without the personal help and guidance of someone who is thoroughly versed in this method of Spiritual training the student should not venture beyond the time of sixteen, sixty-four, thirty-two (seconds). The time value now is usually set by simply counting slowly to the number of seconds chosen, or one may use his Mantra which has been given him by his Guru.

3

The highest practice, Uttama Pranayama, brings the subject to the point where he can do aerial suspension by merely resting the toes or finger-tips on the floor. In time he will be able to rise from the ground without touching anything, and he will be able to bound about like an inflated rubber ball. There are special practices which will enable him to walk on water and do similar feats.

One school of spiritual seekers practises Pranayama by inhaling generously in such a manner as to make it impossible to hear one's breath ; then, after suspending for 120 counts, exhaling in a like manner. The count is gradually increased. The aim is to develop such control over the exhalation that one would not make a candle flame flicker or make an impression on a mirror if it were held beneath the nostrils. One must abstain from the five grains: hempseed, millet seed, corn, rice, and pulse. This method demands steady practice, also that one embrace a number of mental and moral conditions. One must have the right aim and be ready to carry it out and one must be equipped with the proper ideas about the world and the significance of Life. He must face the facts of existence and grasp the first Truth, the Universal Illusion. It is essential to have the right point of view to sustain one in the needful detachment from all sensual desires and to produce a temper of kindness and benevolence.

Breath forced into the arteries of the body is done by Kumbhaka. As it enters the blood it warms the body; it gives a sort of magical warmth and an ecstatic giddiness. The heat produced by Pranayama burns out certain elements of desire, just as a fire burns away chaff. It makes the Yogi free from any transgression of Divine Law and destroys his bonds.

When sufficient heat is gathered, Prana acquires enough strength to affect the mental coil. As long as the cardiac temperature is not strong enough to affect the mental coil, the dreaming state is maintained. It is by the control of Prana that the internal heat (Agni) is increased and with this increase food is easily digested. When food is properly digested there is an increase of the nourishing essence (Rasa). All evil tendencies and diseases now having been consumed, there is an increase in Wisdom. By constant practice the student can gain control in six months. Then his Wayu will enter the middle channel of the body (Sushumna) which gives him control over the mind, and enables him to attain success in this world.

4

Would the day ever come, I wondered, when I could attest to all these mysterious claims and pronounce the Truth of which my teacher spoke? I did not reflect long on its goal of eternal happiness, for I knew my joy would come from getting into action. I was impatient to begin my discipline. Since everything was packed, we lingered a short while after the evening meal, talking about the Swamaji who had initiated me. He had gone to visit, with his old teacher, a Maharishi, who had his retreat hidden away in the hills of Central India. My friend told me that this Holy Man, who was an accomplished Yogi, had been a disciple of my early Guru who had instructed me in America, and that it was planned to have him guide my future discipline. My first teacher on parting from this life had requested that his closest disciple aid me to continue my instruction. Apparently my first Guru had told him a great deal about me and my sincere desire to learn of those teachings as well as live in accordance with its laws. The Swamaji had left word that my Tantrik friend was to bring me to the hermitage of the Maharishi when I returned from my trip.

A teacher, however, will not accept a student until he has first carefully examined him. He must fully determine the student's capacity in order to know what method should be followed. Afterwards the young disciple must pass through a simple initiation, in order that the teacher may establish a psychic bond with his subconscious. The Guru is then able to assist the initiate in his efforts to bring his mind to complete rest and thereby help him along the Path of Inner Understanding.

This conscious tie between them makes it possible for the teacher to be aware at all times of the development attained by the disciple. Even though much of this training was becoming second nature to me, I found a glow still came over me when I contemplated undertaking the discipline with a Guru who had been trained by the teacher that guided my footsteps for so many years.

There was little time to dwell on my feelings, for we had to be up at four, in order to catch the train for Calcutta.

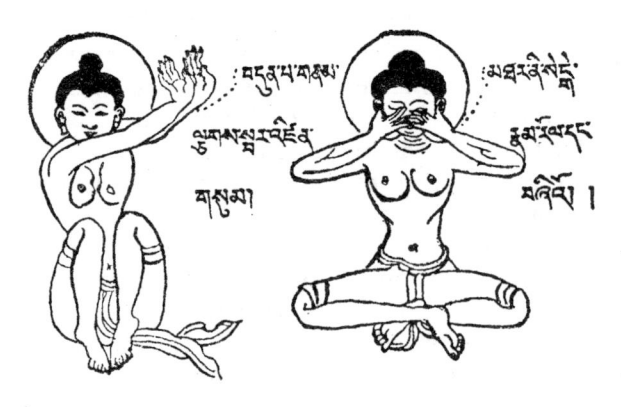

CHAPTER XIV

CONTRASTS IN INDIA

I

WE arrived in Calcutta the following morning about seven, allowing us ample time during the day to do a little shopping and to attend to the minor details of everyday living. That evening, without delay, we were to start for the jungle home of the Maharishi.

An Indian railway station is always teeming with humanity loaded down with countless small bundles, many of which are borne upon the heads of coolies, who dash in and out of the swarming host, their red shirt-tails flapping in the breeze they stir. Frequently they wear a band on their arms on which are inscribed the words, "One Anna," which is the price they are supposed to charge per bundle; actually you always pay two. We travelled Inter-Class, which sometimes permits one to stretch out for a nap, if there is any space left.

Fortunately, we had the Inter-Class car to ourselves, and enjoyed complete privacy. What more could one wish? And it was a car which ordinarily accommodated fourteen persons, if they all sat up. On one side of the car were small wooden benches, all stationary and arranged in one direction and placed crosswise with the car, as in one of our large buses. Against the opposite wall there was constructed a narrow wooden bench running the whole length of the car as in some of our old-fashioned tram-cars but not nearly so comfortable ; the seats were unpadded. You sat on plain wood, with your back to the window.

When travelling in India, one always carries his bedding with him, regardless of the class he uses. By this time I was hardened to riding in Indian trains and never bothered about bedding. I carried only a small blanket in which to roll up in order to keep off a little of the dust. It is worse in India in a train than driving through a dust storm in America. The blanket made it a little easier to throw off what gathered during the night. On this particular occasion I had all my things with me, as I was planning to live in the jungle for an extended period. My entire bed roll provided the luxury of a pillow, so I planned to be really comfortable for one night.

In about an hour we stopped and two fellows joined us. Always a good sleeper, I took the place at the end of the bench, letting my legs, from the knees down, extend over the edge. This had the advantage of allowing me to spread my legs and thus maintain my balance and avoid being shaken off during the night.

About two o'clock I was awakened by a stir of great confusion. I found the car packed to the very limit with people. I counted twenty-six passengers packed in like subway commuters at five o'clock in New York. Since I was awake I got up and went into the small wash room. When I returned the small space I had formerly occupied was taken by a stranger. It seemed to me that passengers seeing the car crowded to the limit might have found accommodations in other coaches on the train, but Indian-like they pack in like animals, being perfectly satisfied to sit for hours so closely packed as to be unable to move. In this particular instance, I was not given to allow myself to be included in such a mode of travel ; so I insisted on having the small space that I had formerly occupied before leaving for the wash room. I asked the chap to move over. He tried to indicate he could not speak English, but this had no effect on me. It was a usual dodge. I simply sat down on the half-inch of space left and gave a forceful shove and another and another until I had made a place for myself. I then informed the fellow that I had been sleeping there and as there wasn't the slightest reaction, I tossed my pillow in his lap and lay down to sleep again. Since he would not move I felt he could hold my head for the night. Soon I felt him sliding out from beneath my weight, so I turned my face to the wall and went to sleep. But not for long. I was presently awakened by someone tugging at my shirt.

After some consideration I turned around. A man in uniform was standing next to me and he started off in typical Indian fashion, asking if I was not ashamed of myself for taking the poor man's seat and crowding him completely out of the car. Here was I, a white man, taking advantage of a poor humble soul, he continued on and on. I became enraged and almost reacted as I had been accustomed to do in the West, where action was the quickest manner of settling such matters. But it flashed in my mind that a white man must never hit a native, no matter what the provocation. So I controlled myself and began to explain that I had boarded the train at the place of origin and since I held a through ticket was privileged to my place. The man in uniform insisted I was not speaking the truth and that the poor soul had been sitting there before me and I usurped his place. I continued to explain, but all in vain. My gorge was rising again.

Finally he insisted he could prove I was wrong if I would get up. I did. He then dug down beneath my pillow along the place where I had been lying and pulled out several things which belonged to the Indian who had placed them there after I had fallen off to sleep. This was going too far. I exploded and told the conductor in no uncertain terms that if that old fellow had to sit or sleep on top of someone there were enough of his own race and kind around; he wasn't forced to pick on a foreigner. While we continued our heated argument, we happened to see the Indian in question crawl in with some of the others. So the conductor had to give up in the end. The train stopped again in about half an hour and every soul got off, except my Tantrik friend and myself. For the remainder of the night we had the car to ourselves. Such is night travel in India in Inter-Class.

2

We left the train the following afternoon and had a couple of cups of tea in a small whitewashed station. Word had been sent ahead so we found that a bullock cart had been sent to meet us. The jungle retreat of the Maharishi whom we were going to visit was situated at a considerable distance from the train line. He did not like to be disturbed in his work by modernity.

There was a long wobbly journey ahead, so we hastened to make a start. A bullock cart travels too slowly to permit one to walk, so the only way to endure this sort of travel is to crawl in on the bed of straw and relax. We had been so long on the train, however, we decided to try walking. No matter how slowly we strolled, we were always ahead of the cart.

Late in the afternoon we arrived at a small Indian village where we were supposed to stop and have a light meal at the home of a native and wait for the bullock cart with our luggage to catch up with us.

It was in the cool of the evening when we set out again and we spent the night snatching what little sleep we could from time to time in the joggling cart, as it squeaked its way along the uneven road. It was a brilliant night; we were travelling in the full of the moon. With my imagination running the gauntlet of dreams, it was quite impossible to think of relaxing. With every jolt, a new idea seemed to spring into my consciousness; I had to strain every effort to keep my mind on the opportunity that was to be offered me, and to plan accordingly. I was on the verge of the realization of my early dreams.

We arrived just as the sun rose into the early morning mist; it hung there like an immense ball of fire. The servants had been up for hours, and were prepared for our arrival. We were promptly escorted to our respective rooms, and presently the much-needed bath water was brought to us.

From the instant I stepped across the threshold of the small room that was to be my home for the next few months it became my sanctuary. To discard my European clothes, to bathe, and then put on my Dhoti (the cloth worn by the native), gave me the feeling of being born into a new world. Seven or eight yards in length, the Dhoti is wrapped around the waist to fit like a diaper; arranged like a pair of pants, the insides of the legs are left almost completely bare, allowing the breezes to play on the skin. An ordinary shirt, with the collar unbuttoned and the shirt-tail hanging down outside, drapes the upper portion of the body. It is by far the most comfortable way to dress. Not only is it cool, but it permits much freedom of action, especially when one is sitting cross-legged, according to the custom.

In one corner of the room, on the floor, was a low wooden platform, covered with a mat. It was to serve the purposes of a bed. I was not only to sleep here, but also to do all of my work. It was oblong in shape, and large enough to let me have considerable freedom of action, for it was here that I would do all my practices, and it was also to become my shrine; once I had consecrated this corner, thenceforward no one else would touch it. Next to the wall opposite this corner there was a small mat spread on the floor; it was a place for a visitor to sit. Close to my own mat was a small box, upon which I placed my typewriter; it also was to serve as a chest for my private papers. Apart from this one piece of furniture, there was not another thing in the room. The walls had been recently whitewashed, and gave me a feeling of immaculate cleanliness. The bed was so placed as to permit me to sleep north and south. Just over my shoulder was a window which would provide adequate light for all of my studies during the day, when I was not engaged in my practices. A short way from the window, at the foot of my bed, was a door leading into a small outer room which served as a bathroom, providing the customary native facilities but little different from those of the backwoods of our own country a hundred years ago.

I had few belongings apart from books, but of these I had a sizable collection. Some of them were rare. I had collected most of them in the course of my travels. They were always with me, as a very essential part of my being, inseparable from me. I arranged them for ready access in my suit-cases.

3

After I had had my bath, I walked out into a large compound that surrounded the small cloister, which consisted of several other rooms like the one allotted to me. Two of the rooms were being used by my Tantrik friend and the Swamaji who had initiated me, while some of the other rooms were used by the attendants. Behind the open compound was a large building occupied by the servants; in its proximity was the kitchen. The Maharishi, under whose guidance I was to take up my discipline, had his small hermitage a few minutes' walk from here. In the middle of this compound was a tree with a low wall built around it to allow one to sit in its shade. I sat here for some time, pondering on what was yet to happen to me. Would I be the same when I left this place?

The servants soon called me to breakfast, which was being served in a room set aside for the purpose when guests were around. This was the first time that I had seen the Swamaji since my return. He was greatly interested in hearing about my Indian travels and in what I had been able to learn in my contacts. It was necessary for me to review my entire experience again.

The Swamaji had come here to carry on some research work in Tantrik chemistry, for the Maharishi was reputed to have a vast knowledge of this subject. He said he could not continue much longer, as he was running out of supplies. My Tantrik friend and he, however, would be around long enough to see to it that I was fully under way with my practice. By then I would no longer need an interpreter. They pointed out that as soon as the Maharishi had initiated me, it would not matter whether or no he could talk to me, for he would not know exactly what was going on inside of me all the time. They spoke of the Maharishi with a reverence that was inspiring.

The person who had been selected by this Holy Man to take care of his daily necessities of living (such as preparing and serving food, etc.) was a man of considerable learning who could speak a little English. These Holy Men are very strict as to who is chosen to care for them and prepare their food. The ordinary servant is not permitted to come into their sanctuaries. I was to be an added burden and responsibility for the Maharishi's personal attendant who also was assigned to take care of me.

It is the usual experience of persons from the West who go to India to find that the ordinary servants have little mental capacity and are unreliable to an extreme. It can be very trying to see that he does everything right, so it was a great relief to me to be able to turn over all the minor cares of living to a high-class Brahmin who would prepare my food and see to it that the servants attended to their duties. This would permit me to devote every second to my studies and to the discipline that I was to undergo.

4

Shortly after lunch we took a five minutes' walk over a well-trodden path to the Maharishi's hermitage. His sanctuary consisted of a small compound that was full of seasonal flowers. There were not many in bloom at this time but all was green. The entrance to his small retreat was covered by a dense growth of vines which gave shade and protection against the intense sun. It was a brick building of native manufacture, rather long and narrow, divided into three sections. The first was his private room where he lived and carried on all his practices. The second had a small shrine. The last was probably used as a storeroom.

No sooner had we entered the gate of the compound than his attendant came to welcome us. It was a matter of only a minute or so before we were escorted into his private room. As each of us stepped across the threshold we kneeled before him, placing our heads and folded hands on his feet. He blessed us with a touch of his hands. Some lovely mats had been placed on the floor for us and some Indian sweets were brought in and left within our reach so we might nibble as we talked.

It took a few minutes for me to become accustomed to the dim light of the room, which contained only one small window. Next to the window was a wooden bed which was covered with a tiger skin on which it is customary for every Holy Man to have his seat. His body was covered with a shawl of reddish cloth, which indicated his rank. His face was lighted with a smile which did not cause a wrinkle. His eyes sparkled and seemed to peer right into the depths of your consciousness. His tonsured head was almost luminous. His posture was erect but completely relaxed and he spoke with a clear, soft, melodious tone of voice that held your attention even though you could not understand what he said.

Through my interpreters I expressed my appreciation of the privilege he had granted by accepting me. It was going to mean a great deal to me to be able to continue my work under the guidance of one who had been a disciple of my first Guru, who had recently passed away.

He told me that my first Guru had spoken to him about me and that he had been waiting for ever so long a time to meet me because of the faith my first teacher had in me. He had been watching my studies and efforts with great interest, he continued, and then asked questions as to how I was enjoying my trip to India aside from my studies. He wanted to know if I was lonesome for all I had left behind.

My Tantrik friend took up the conversation and related my experiences, the progress in my studies, and, I presume, added his private opinion of me. He knew more about me than anyone else.

Before we left we got into a philosophical discussion of the need of understanding the philosophy behind the practices in order to gain the inner benefit from them. The practices, after all, are only the means to an end —but they are the only means. It is necessary that one rub out the mind, and the mind cannot do anything without the practices. Knowledge is only an accessory to the end and not the true pathway, for the end cannot be attained by head work alone. A philosophical understanding is essential to fortify one in the rigid discipline of the practices.

The Maharishi said that many of my letters had been read to him and that he was certain I was prepared and that he would choose an auspicious day for my initiation. In the meantime I was to prepare myself for this day. He said no more, but I could see what he meant. This was going to be his way of discovering what I really did know.

I found a deep inner peace in just being allowed to sit in his presence. There was something so mysterious yet simple, so divinely magnetic about him, that the flames of inspiration within became almost out of control. I was deeply moved. What a heaven on this earth it would be if there were places in the midst of the bustling, strident Western activity where those who were aspiring to other things could gather together in order to renew their strength in their common understanding and desire ! This was my opportunity to taste of the joys that can be found if one can even temporarily live with an individual whose life is being directed and guided by the true purpose of human existence.

Every hour was an inspiration, and every activity pointed to the one goal of Spiritual Growth. To be able just to sit and listen to them talk, even though I could not understand one word, was a source of much inner strength. I was so lost within myself it seemed only a few seconds before we had to leave so that the Maharishi could continue his discipline.

I was too much lost in the flood of emotions to do anything for the rest of the afternoon, so I explored a few of the neighbouring trails in order to choose one for my daily walk. This is the way to relax between periods of practice. I had noted that the Maharishi had a short path, about 150 feet in length, over which he would stroll for relaxation. This is a technique which is often used by Holy Men who confine themselves a great deal. They do much of their reflecting in this manner. So I chose mine. I knew I ought to choose the one I liked best, for I should not wish to change. One grows accustomed to one's path; he comes to know the varied contours of the rocks and almost the individual blades of grass beside it. Then he dislikes giving it up and establishing this intimacy with another.

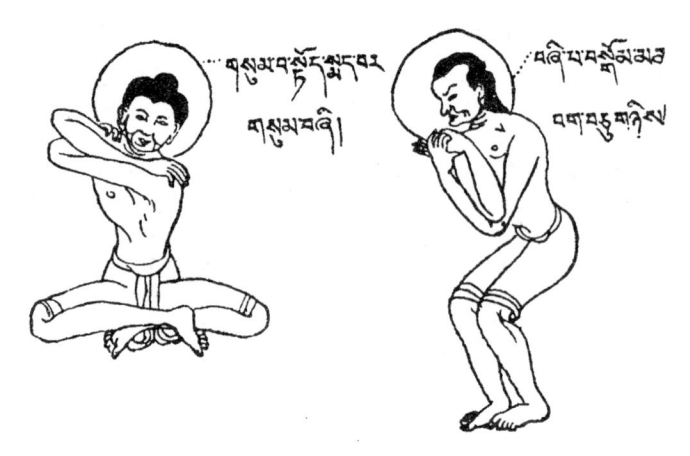

CHAPTER XV

IMPORTANT POSTURES IN YOGA

I

THAT evening after dinner the Swamaji, my Tantrik friend, and myself entered into a brief discussion about the Asanas (postures) which one must perfect in his early Yoga training. I brought up the subject because I knew the time had come when I must perfect all the basic Asanas. The Swamaji pointed out that the root meaning of Asana is to become master, to enjoy, to reach across; that there are as many postures as there are numbers of species of living creatures in the Universe. Out of eighty-four special postures thirty-two have been selected as most useful to mankind. These are given in the Gheranda Samhita, which is an authoritative text of Yoga, and for purposes of reference I list them here: Siddhasana, Padmasana, Bhadrasana, Muktasana, Vajrasana, Swastikasana, Simhasana, Gomukhasana, Virasana, Dhanurasana, Mritasana, Guptasana, Matsyasana, Matsyendrasana, Goraksasana, Pashchimottanasana, Utkatasana, Samkatasana, Mayurasana, Kukkutsana, Kurmasana, Uttana Kurmakasana, Uttana Mandukasana, Vrikshasana, Mandukasana. Garudasana, Vrishana, Shalabhasana, Makarasana, Ushtrasana, Bhujangasana, and Yogasana.

He continued to explain that Asanas are the first accessories to Hatha Yoga, and sixteen of them are essential in order to complete its practices, while four of them are of special importance. These four are: Siddhasana, Padmasana, Swastikasana, and Vajrasana.

Postures are practised to equalize and still bodily forces, to control circulation and respiration, and to bring the spine to its natural curve. The production of carbonic acid gas in the system is reduced by the reduction of the internal activities of the body, which also causes a proportional reduction in the expenditure of energy during the time that the pose is maintained. The heart action becomes slower, and gradually one feels that one scarcely has a body. Delivered from the awareness of physical conditions, the mind can engage in meditation for lengthy periods.

Asanas have no specific action on the arteries; some of them, however, help the veins. Various postures are essential to general health, while others secure one an immunity from diseases, calm the passions, give peace of mind, and enable the Yogi to attend to his ambitions. It is proven that if certain positions of the body are assumed and held for certain lengths of time, and breathing exercises practised, different effects will result in accordance with the postures.

There is not a single posture which does not indirectly lead to spiritual progress. Some directly help to arouse spiritual forces. Two classifications of the Asanas, however, are made: spiritual and physical. The latter sort are used for the purpose of establishing a balance in the various physiological functions of the body so that its energies may possess the ultimate organic vigour. Chief of these are Sirshasana, Sarvangasana, and Halasana.

The principal spiritual Asanas intended to aid one in the process of abstraction, concentration, meditation, and trance are: Siddhasana, Padmasana, Swastikasana, and Sukhasana.

2

In the *Vedanta Sara* it is said that at the time of lying down, rising, or moving about, one's mind is agitated. Therefore these poses are essential for concentration. If a man lies down at the time of meditation he may fall asleep, if he stands there will be agitation of mind; both of these are obviously impediments to meditation. The poses cause freedom of the abdominal viscera, a reduction in the generation of carbon dioxide gas to a minimum so that the respiration may become imperceptible, a toning of the coccygeal and sacral nerves, thus supplying a rich and abundant quantity of blood to the pelvic region where the static background of man's powers reside.

One of the aims of Yoga is to train the will power. A steady posture must not be neglected if the student wishes to bring both his body and mind under the domination of his will. One of the most helpful steps in all mind training is the ability to forget the body at will. This can be accomplished by the Asanas. Only when the body is kept under subjection do the desires come under control. When the desires are under control, the mind is indirectly controlled.

Asanas are a primary prerequisite to either physical or mental development. They not only bring about a steadiness of body and mind; they are also pleasant to practise. Yoga requires that the student take a particular pose and maintain it without any movement for a specified time. Siddhasana and Padmasana are the chief postures. Siddhasana should come first. Once accomplished it should continue to be practised. The lower extremities of the body must form a fixed base and the upper portion of the body should always be held erect. Eventually the mind will become free from any burden of the body and lose all consciousness of it.

Steadiness, calmness, and the cessation of activity of Prana do not manifest themselves without posture. When the body is at rest, the vital forces do not stream through it, therefore breathing is quiet and the mind finds no obstructions. In the perfected pose, which is one sustained for three hours, the breath is motionless and the mind and body become one.

Certain poses are calculated to bring a rich supply of blood to the brain and to the various parts of the spine, directly benefiting the brain, the spinal cord, and the sympathetic nervous system. Sirshasana supplies the brain, Halasana supplies the dorsal and lumbar region of the spine. Padmasana and Pashchimottanasana supply the lumbar and sacral regions, Mayurasana supplies the upper lumbar and dorsal section of the spinal column by mechanically checking the abdominal aorta before it bifurcates in front of the fourth lumbar vertebra. Other Asanas were evolved to stretch and bend the spine in various ways, much as if it were massaged. This promotes the health of the nerves which are rooted therein and develops the vertebral column in the most effective way.

A sort of pad or cushion about the dimensions of a bed covered with a white cloth is generally used as one's seat in performing the various postures. A pad of this size is essential because some of the postures are done while lying prone. For the purpose of meditation, however, and for most of the Pranayama practices a soft but firm seat about two feet square, made of sheep skin or tiger skin, or a folded woollen blanket or silk-covered cushion may be used.

3

The beginner must ponder on such matters as Self-investigation and Self-control. This means pondering upon sincerity. One must constantly be drilling oneself to perfect each step, never overlooking anything because it appears to be inconsequential. It requires deliberate effort to regulate the body and thereby rectify the mind. It is essential to withdraw from all passions or else give way to them and thus rid the mind of them.

For the purpose of meditation, Siddhasana or Padmassana must be developed to the point where it is possible to hold it from one-half to one hour, at the least. There can be no meditation without it. As explained, it is essential that the body and breath become quiescent for meditation. There must be complete accord of the physical with the mental. In the beginning effort should be devoted to the pose which is most agreeable, practising steadily with the aim of finally accomplishing Padmasana. Padmasana is important because it can be used for all purposes and is absolutely essential in some instances. The other Asanas may be developed slowly with the object of keeping the body fully flexed and aiding general physical efficiency and symmetry.

Since it is possible to find descriptions of all these Asanas in other texts, I will here describe only the four most important ones.

Siddhasana is called the Perfect posture or the pose of the adept. Siddha means adept in Sanskrit. It is the Asana for both Pranayama and mind control and can be developed very easily by almost anyone.

In a sitting position, stretch out the legs and then bend the left leg at the knee joint, folding it upon itself and placing the heel tightly against the perineum. The sole of the left foot should be touching the upper portion of the thigh. No attempt should be made to sit upon the heel. The pressure is exerted on the perineum, not the anus. The adjusted heel should feel the touch of the bones on the two sides of the perineum. The genitals are now arranged within the space of the left thigh and the left calf. The right leg should now be folded after the same manner, placing its heel against the pubic bone just above the sex organ. The right foot should spread along the left thigh, the lower border of the foot being thrust between the left thigh and the left calf. The spine must be kept erect. The hands may be placed upon the knees. This is the usual position in meditation.

On the other hand, the right hand may be placed

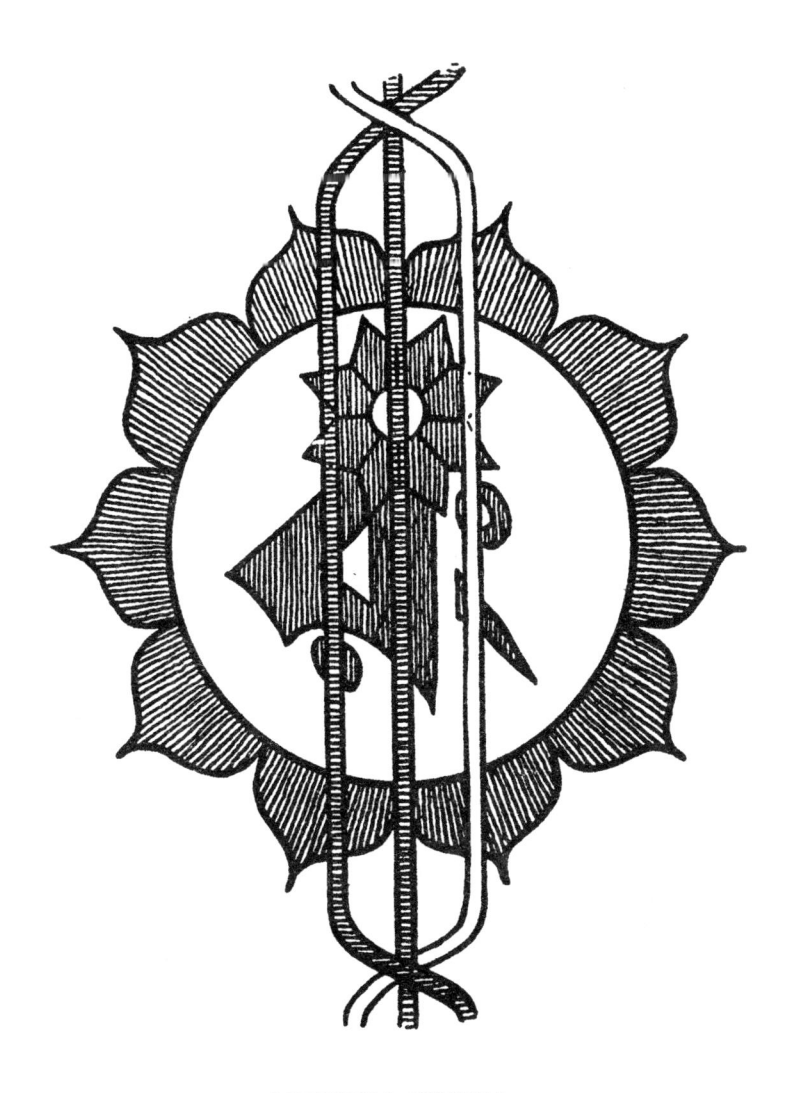

MANIPURA CHAKRA

upon the right thigh and the left hand upon the left thigh, or the arms extended with the wrists resting upon the knee, the palms open and directed upward, the tip of the index finger of each hand touching the tip of the respective thumb, the rest of the fingers fully extended. The chin is placed in the jugular notch. The eyes are made to gaze steadily on the space between the eyebrows.

Siddhasana is an instrument for the freeing of one from the miseries of this world. It opens the door to salvation. If this pose is done under the precepts of Yoga it will restore the loss of vital power, disease will disappear, and magical powers will be developed.

If this Asana is difficult at first, the student may take up Swastikasana, which will be found easier and more simple. It will provide practice until the more difficult Asanas can be performed.

Padmasana is known as the Lotus posture and is considered to be foremost of all the Asanas. Since it has already been described, only its fully developed form will be given here. Its perfected form is known as Wadda Padmasana. After sitting in Padmasana, the student is to cross his arms behind him so that it will be possible for him to take hold of the great toe of the right foot with the right hand from behind his back and the great left toe with the left hand after the same manner. The best way to develop the practice is to extend one arm around the back and grip its wrist with the other hand and pull, in such a manner that it will bring the hand as far forward as possible. By changing from one arm to the other it will soon flex the shoulders and arms so that it will be possible to execute this practice. Those who cannot cross their arms behind their back to obtain a hold on the feet may place the palm of the left hand under the right foot and the right hand under the left foot.

After assuming the pose, Jalandhara (chin lock) is done and the eyes are centred on the tip of the nose which tends to quiet the movement of the eyes and to

Important Postures in Yoga

suspend the activity of the mind. This enables one to observe the rise of the Tattwas as well as those fine offshoots of light from both Ida and Pingala that go before the eyes. In crossing the arms behind the back and tightly locking them with the hold on the feet, a pressure is placed on the armpits which directly affects Ida and Pingala. The heel pressure in the groins and the pressure beneath the knee joints check the lower circuit of Ida and Pingala. Everything in the pose has a tendency to calm the flow of these two breaths which then enables Sushumna to work.

This leads to a positive control of the mind. One should sit calmly, restraining all sense, and never permitting sleep to overcome one when in this pose. When this pose is perfected and Pranayama perfected all diseases will disappear. Kundalini will be awakened and freedom from all bondage and the highest intelligence will result.

It must be understood that where such comments as this are made on the effects of a practice, it is presumed that a full course of Yoga has been completed. These are end results.

Swastikasana is known as the Prosperous posture, also as the easy pose. It is accomplished by first taking one's place upon the floor with legs outstretched. Then bend the right leg at the knee and fold as in Siddhasana, but instead of placing the heel against the perineum, set the foot against the opposite groin so that the sole is in close contact with the opposite thigh. Then, without disturbing the position of the heel, raise the toes of the right foot with the left hand, simultaneously folding the left leg and placing the left foot against the right groin and thigh. The big toe of the right foot should project above the calf and thigh, between which it is held, the heel being firmly set against the right groin. The toes of the left foot should then be inserted between the right calf and right thigh, allowing only the left big toe to project. The legs should be crossed just above the ankles so that all unpleasant pressure on the bones can be avoided. If the student prefers he may start with the left leg.

The palms are placed upon the knees or the arms may be placed out a little farther, in which case the hands are placed as in Siddhasana, or the hands should rest upon the heels with the palms turned upwards. In the latter position the back of the left hand should touch the heels and the right hand should then be set in the left hand.

The spine must be kept erect. The eyes must be kept closed, while one practises the Nasal or Frontal gaze.

Swastikasana is a meditative pose. It should be practised until it can be maintained for a considerable length of time. In this pose the pelvic region gets a large supply of blood, the coccygeal and sacral nerves are toned and the flow of Ida and Pingala is somewhat arrested. Then Wayu Siddhi (control over the air) is easily obtained.

Vajrasana is known as the Thunderbolt posture. This is primarily a meditative pose ; its physical advantages are inconsiderable.

It is accomplished by taking one's seat with the legs extended. One leg is flexed at the knee joint and the foot brought back to the buttock on that side. This buttock is then raised, the trunk inclining a little to the opposite side, supported by the hand on that side. The foot which is now at the buttock is drawn slightly to the side and extended so that the sole is upturned, the knee being lowered to the floor. The toes are arranged behind the slightly raised buttock and the heel is now in the clear. The other leg is then put through the same régime. In the final stage one's seat is between the two feet on the floor, the feet forming a sort of curve around the buttocks. The toes are directed toward each other with the heels upturned. The knees lie together, the spine is held erect, the eyes are kept closed, the palms cover the knees. The pose is now complete.

Another arrangement is the Japanese manner of sitting. Instead of keeping the legs clear of the thighs and buttocks, they are placed underneath the latter so that the student sits upon his ankles, the two sets of toes crossing behind the lower spine, the knees lying close together. When properly seated, the spine is drawn erect, the palms placed upon the knees and the eyes closed.

Students who find their joints stiff and who cannot get down on the floor in this manner should proceed with extreme caution. The joints should be flexed again and again while supporting the body by holding to something firm and only when the joints have required the necessary suppleness should the student attempt the full pose. One should practise twice daily, starting with a few minutes and gradually increasing the time of each practice. The circulation in the lower extremities is very much checked and the lower trunk is abundantly supplied with fresh and freely circulating blood. This pose is used for spiritual purposes in Yoga Training.

A further development of this pose is known as Supta Vajrasana, or Supine Pelvic Pose. Instead of sitting erect, the trunk is inclined until it rests supine upon the floor. This, of course, must be done slowly. The practice must be extended over a long period so that undue strain is not put on the muscles and tendons. Reclining backwards, the trunk is supported by the hands. Then one hand is removed and the weight on that side thrown upon the elbow. The same is then done on the other side. Then, one at a time, both elbows are removed and the body rests upon the shoulder blades. The curve of the trunk lessens and finally it becomes straight in contact with the seat. There is considerable strain on the ankles and caution must be observed.

Next lift the head and place the forearms under it crosswise. They will serve as a cushion for the head. The hands grasp the shoulders on the opposite sides, the two elbows projecting a little beyond the head. The eyes are closed.

In coming out of the pose the hands must be released first or it may result in injury to the ankles. The action of this pose is more accentuated than in Vajrasana. It has a specific effect on the pelvic organs and the abdominal wall and viscera are stimulated considerably. It also stretches the nerves that are connected with the function of sex and strengthens them.

4

Our discussion for the evening was finished. In order to be up at four to begin my practice, I must get to bed at a reasonable hour. Now I was to live the life of a Yogi, adhering to the letter of all the regulations of a Yogi's daily life. This meant that I must gradually reduce the hours of sleep, but the first night was no time to begin.

My friends were pleased at my eagerness to take up the practices and were anxious to do everything they could for me. But, as they pointed out, the work was up to me. They could guide and instruct, but only by practice can anyone become an accomplished Yogi.

Early tea was to be omitted and in no circumstances was I to be disturbed before eight o'clock, when I might have honey, barley meal, and hot milk. I had to smile when I realized that it would be necessary for me to break every rule of living that had been given me in the United States. My doctor and friends had cautioned me about drinking milk in the Orient, or eating fruit or vegetables unless they were first thoroughly cleansed with potassium permanganate.

Obviously it was impossible to follow this advice. I had come here to live as a disciple. It was their claim their practices would absolutely free one from all diseases.

I had to have Faith.

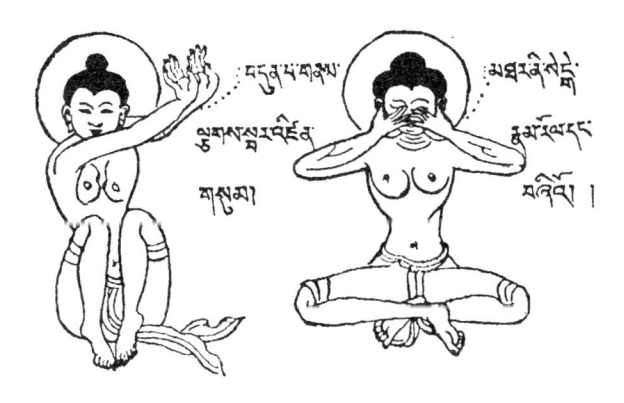

CHAPTER XVI

STANDING ON ONE'S HEAD, ETC.

I

I HAD scarcely sunk into sleep, when four o'clock came and I had to be up. Promptly I set to work to do Dhauti, which, if you will recall, is the swallowing of a long piece of cloth for the purpose of thoroughly cleansing the stomach and removing all excess Kapha. This exercise has also a stimulating effect on certain important nerve centres.

I followed this with Neti. Instead of running the string up through the nostrils and bringing it out through the mouth, I used the water method, which consists of sucking water up through the nostrils and spitting it out, and of then reversing the process by drawing the water up through the mouth and expelling it through the nostrils. This cleans and enlivens the nerve centres in the head.

It had been a regular practice of mine for a long period to stretch the tongue, so that I might perform Khecari, or the swallowing of the tongue, an exercise which it was necessary to master before I could take up the advanced Pranayama practices. I devoted some fifteen minutes to this exercise.

By now it was a quarter to five, for I had lost some time in the washing and cleaning of my cloth after doing Dhauti. I was alive to the need of sterilizing everything; it was a reminder from my Western past. Yet sterilization on the Occidental plan was out of the question. Instead, I used a small bucket of water that had been brought from the well that served the compound, and this had to suffice. In the beginning I quailed at the possible outcome of my risk; yet for the reader's peace of mind, I am in a position to assure him that I did not contract any of the diseases which are so prevalent in the Orient.

I had been keeping up the practice of Uddiyana for some years; so I found no difficulty in doing the exercise 1500 times. This would usually occupy me for about half an hour. Then I would devote fifteen minutes to Nauli, which is the isolation of the recti muscles, so that they may be rolled in all directions.

By this time I had made some inroads into the day; certainly, nothing could be more effective for opening one's sleepy eyes than the practices I have just mentioned. The only difficult moment is that in which one must summon courage to make the first jump out of bed.

In order to prepare for my initiation, it was necessary for me to bring all the cleansing practices up to their maximum standard. I had already perfected all of the rudimentary practices during my years of training in America; it was now only a matter of putting them all together as a set of exercises. I had been told of the psychological effect they would have in time, and now it was all confirmed in my personal experience. I had only to perform them to their maximum standard for awhile, and I would be not only physically ready but also spiritually awake to receive what my Guru was going to pass on to me. I had maintained my Yogic discipline all those years in order to be ready to carry on my work under a teacher, and now I felt that the labours had not been in vain. I was, in any event, conscious of the awakening of all the psychic forces of my body. And, indeed, the next eight or ten days were to be a period of a spiritual tuning up.

2

A quarter of six I set as the time to begin standing on my head for half an hour. Having already brought up this practice to its maximum standard of three hours, I found no difficulty in resuming the practice for a mere half-hour, even though I had not practised it for a few months. It was, in fact, the one practice that I had missed most during the months of abstention; in many respects, I have never found its equal. In it, it is possible to experience a peace of relaxation unavailable in any other form. Yet, from my own experience, I must caution everyone to proceed slowly in developing this practice. Among other things this exercise is the best indication of the condition of the body. One must be in the finest health in order to receive its benefits rather than its burdens. Indeed, it must be stressed that it involves not a little danger if one is not thoroughly cleansed and the body is functioning imperfectly. It is, however, the perfect exercise for those in perfect condition. All others must beware.

It is a relatively simple matter to find one's capacity in this or in any other practice of Yoga. When you first go up on your head, you will experience a feeling of complete relaxation, but as you begin to approach your capacity you will inevitably feel a nervous tension creeping over the body; this will manifest itself in a desire to wiggle, to kick your legs, to move them in all directions. Your mind will, at the same time, begin to wander; you will become very time-conscious and will want to look at your timepiece every ten seconds or so, under the impression that several minutes have passed. Small beads of perspiration will begin to break out all over the body. It is time to stop. Check yourself, for you may have reached your capacity, beyond which you should not try to strive. By daily practice, however, you will find that ultimately these distressing manifestations will subside. Then only, when you have attained a peace and have become utterly unaware of the passage of time, will you realize that you have reached a point when you try to increase the effort a trifle, until you begin to sense the approaching nervous tension; then hold on for a bit. It is always advisable to stay far within your limits.

I had tested myself before beginning this practice, and found that I could do it comfortably for an hour. As, henceforth, I was to adhere to it regularly over an extended period of time, it was best to cut my limit in half, so that I would be certain of succeeding. Nothing was to be gained, I knew, by continuing for a full hour and then never be able to do it again. I would accomplish a great deal more if I could hold to a schedule over a period of months; I was playing safe. I wanted results, regardless of how small they might be.

On finishing the head stand, I began my Pranayama practice. Eventually, I would devote most of the time to this practice, whose purpose was to provide the key to the Yogic way of life, but for this one must be in perfect condition, if results are to be achieved. With time, I would be increasing the periods spent on this practice, and decreasing the periods spent on the purification practices.

In the beginning, Pranayama would serve as a gauge of my progress with the cleansing practices; it would provide a kind of measuring-stick for checking up on my other work.

I began my Pranayama practice at six-thirty sharp, after practising a few of the simple cleansing breaths to prepare me for it.

I assumed Padmasana (the Lotus Pose) in the corner in which I carried on all my work. This was a means of doing two things at one and the same time. I had long made it a practice of doing all of my work in the cross-legged position, so that the limbs might gradually become flexible enough to enable me to do all the required Asanas. Then, too, I knew that I would be able to gain far better results with my Pranayama as soon

Standing On One's Head, etc.

as it was possible for me to carry on the practice in this position.

I began the practice with Bhastrika, which is a nerve-cleansing exercise that is required of all who intend to take up the practice of Yoga. Due to the fact that I had developed the abdominal muscles to such a high degree, this exercise at the rate of sixty strokes a minute was easy. I found I could do it at the top speed of 120, but because of the ever-present danger of fatigue limited myself to the lower speed and did it for one minute only. I inhaled slowly and as deeply and fully as possible, then suspended for one minute, then exhaled as slowly as possible. This in the beginning consumed two and one-half minutes. My second round began at three minutes, so I did ten rounds in thirty minutes. After one week I lifted the suspension to two minutes. It was my plan to increase my Kumbhaka at the rate of one minute a week until I had reached the first degree of perfection. All practices were aimed at that goal.

I finished that morning at seven o'clock, after three hours of practice. This was to be my daily minimum for the next few months. Everything might vary according to results, of course, and my teacher kept close watch of my practices so that I could be certain of success.

As I had an hour before my breakfast would be brought in, I decided to take a stroll.

Never have I known such deep and abiding joy, such thrills of ecstasy, such a richness of living, as filled me then. I was conscious of every minute aspect of life. My body seemed to be glowing in harmony with all Nature. I had a sense of awareness far beyond anything I can describe. There seemed to be no one thing which set off this spark; it came from my soul's contact with the Universal Flow of Life. My entire system vibrated to the rhythm of Nature.

Great peace and strength come as the dawn and while you are breathless with its passing grandeur, it vanishes. Now I was going to be able to establish at will this contact with the Universal Flow of Life. I would need no sunset flaming over the Arizona Deserts, nor would it be fleeting. I could hold it in my inner consciousness until I drank to satiation and so vitalize my daily life.

This morning I made the contact underneath a tree at the end of my short stroll. I had a view of the surrounding country-side. It was a fleeting experience on this morning, but I knew it would not be long before it would be possible to sustain it much longer. With my daily practice I intended to increase my capacity so that I could store enough in all the tissues of my body to carry me for years to come. My opportunity was at hand. I was going to Drink Deep.

3

After breakfast I studied. It was my plan to study the theory as I practised. This seemed to me essential if I was to teach others who yearned to learn this ageless spiritual science which has been passed down by word of mouth from teacher to pupil for centuries. It is taught that this is the method through which Buddha and Christ both received their enlightenment.

The Truth is changeless; only forms change. Hence it is necessary to discover new forms which will reveal to man his inner self and enable him to contact this eternal stream of life. This made it imperative that I find my way back to the Eternal Truth through the archaic forms of the past, then by living in life I could find this same Truth in the new forms of our Modern Era.

At ten-thirty I resumed my practices, beginning with Khecari which I worked at for fifteen minutes. At a quarter before eleven I stood on my head for thirty minutes. By now I could hold the head stand in the middle of the room without the slightest difficulty.

There is no rule which forbids the beginner to do the head stand against the wall in order better to maintain balance. For a mat on which to rest the head, a large bath towel or blanket, folded several times, is recom-

Standing On One's Head, etc.

mended for the beginner, but I needed nothing more than a normal carpet. After finishing the head stand, I took my seat in the Padmasana position and spent thirty minutes on Pranayama. I always began this exercise with Bhastrika as prescribed.

By this time my body was warm enough to practise the Asanas. It is customary to practise these after everything else has been done, making rather a side issue of them. This is a little trick to overcome the monotony. As the student will discover, in Yoga it is all work and no play.

There were sixteen Asanas which it was necessary for me to develop; some of them, however, were, more or less, combinations of the others. This list of Asanas is common knowledge to all who are familiar with the published literature of Yoga.

It would be sufficient for me to hold Padmasana for a period of three hours, but it was essential that I learn the technique of the others for each and everyone has a specific purpose, and I could never foresee when I would need one of them to overcome some difficulty I might encounter.

Lunch was brought in about one o'clock. This was my only real meal. It consisted of some local vegetables prepared with Ghee (clarified butter) and a couple of glasses of milk. I had always been a heavy eater, but never did I enjoy meals so much as these. This was true even when my diet was eventually reduced to nothing but liquids: two glasses of clarified butter and several glasses of milk per day. This seemed ample and never have I been in better health.

After lunch I reclined for the next hour or so. This period, when the heat was most intense, was usually devoted to reading. It is frequently the practice of Yogi to set aside this time for visitors.

A little after two, I went with my friends to visit again with the Maharishi and tell him of my morning activities. He asked me to show him the different Asanas I had practised. Afterwards, he demonstrated exactly how they should be done. It was an inspiration to watch him assume these intricate postures. He did it with the utmost ease and grace and gave me a clear picture of how they should be executed. He had arrived at a degree of perfection which I shall probably never attain. Ten years of his life had been devoted exclusively to the practice of Asanas. He told me that in his youth he had followed paths which were blind alleys. This was before he was fortunate enough to find a teacher who could properly guide him. At that time, he had thought that the practices and perfection of the Asanas alone would enable him to reach his inner goal. He related this with a twinkle in his eye, telling me there was no one Royal Road. Rather it was a matter of combining many ways with intelligence. Everything varies, of course, according to the individual.

The Maharishi was rather astounded when I told him how many times I had done Uddiyana and Nauli. He pointed out that what I had done was considered to be its perfection. He then asked me to show him just how I had been doing it. Afterwards, he said I was ready to learn Basti, which is a method for internal cleansing. With my capacity, he said it would be only a matter of a day or so before I could do the exercise. Of course, first I had to learn the method.

In order to teach me how to do it he gave me the first exercise which is required to gain control over the rectal muscles. The practice is called Aswini Mudra. At no time would he give end results. Never until I had perfected the step which he had given me, would he give the next.

For clarity here, however, I will relate Aswini Mudra and Basti together in the following chapter.

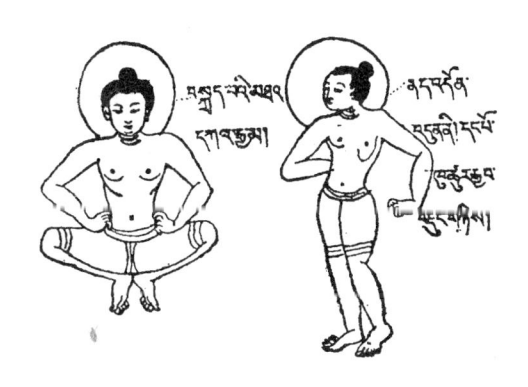

CHAPTER XVII

ABOUT MUDRAS

I

ASWINI MUDRA is a practice to open the rectal muscles. It is one of the most important Mudras. This Mudra may be practised along with Uddiyana to force open the rectum. Considerable work must be done on the anal sphincters, which are the muscles that compress the rectum. First take a position on the elbows and knees, then, after exhaling, pull the navel as far back toward the spine as possible and contract the anal muscles. Try to pull the anus and navel together. While suspending the breath, contract the anus, then relax, trying to push it as far out as possible. Then draw in again. By constant practice of this exercise the student will gain full control over the rectal muscles.

A normal person should gain this control in about two weeks, if one hour a day is given to practice. The result will render it possible to draw in the anus and so relax the sphincters that the gasses which are confined in the colon will be expelled as the abdomen is compressed for Uddiyana.

The Apana gas will not come out so long as there is any water or solid matter in the intestines. As this subtle gas comes from the rectum, it is very cool and there is no sound or odour. The object is to keep it out of the blood. Then one will have control over Apana Wayu.

My teacher pointed out again to me that it is necessary first to perfect Uddiyana and Nauli. With my degree of development he thought I would probably be able to do it almost immediately. When these sphincters come under control and Nauli is done, fresh air will rush into the colon. This gives a sense of lightness and relief.

After some control has been developed, the student should take a squatting position with the buttocks resting on the heels. The rest of the body should sink in between the knees and the arms be locked around them in order to get the needed pressure. Practice in this position should be continued until it is possible to open the sphincters at will. By constant practice in contracting and relaxing the anal aperture, such control can be gained that it is possible to open the rectum and draw water into the colon. This Yogi flushing of the colon is called Basti.

Aswini Mudra stimulates the sympathetic nervous system because the nerve supply of the anus and rectum is mainly connected with the sympathetic nervous system. A large number of nerves end in the mucous membrane of the anal orifice, so this practice gives a definite stimulus to the entire sympathetic system. It is said that Aswini Mudra destroys diseases of the rectum and gives strength and vigour to the entire body. It prevents premature death and assists in the awakening of Kundalini.

2

Mahavadasa Basti is the Yogic method of washing the colon. Basti is practised by the side of a river. The student enters the stream and wades out until the water reaches the navel, when in a squatting position. Then place the feet about a foot apart and proceed to take the squatting position, flexing the knees, rocking forward on the toes, and placing the buttocks on the heels. Rest the forearms on the knees as this gives a good mechanical advantage in the muscular exercise neces-

About Mudras

sary to this practice. The head should be hung down and the spine given a good curve so that, with muscular effort, the essential concave appearance of the abdomen is pronounced.

In the beginning, before the student is able to open his rectum by the practice of Nauli, he is advised to use a hollow piece of bamboo four inches long with a bore of some three-eighths of an inch. Scrape its walls until it is reduced to about three-fifths of an inch in thickness and the two ends well rounded off. Bending slightly forward, the tube, well-lubricated, is introduced to about three-fourths of its length. Then by doing Nauli and holding it as long as possible the water will rush into the colon. When the breath can no longer be held out, the tube is removed and the anal sphincters closed. After a few normal respirations, the student should return to the shore and practise Nauli a few times before he expels the water. If he has any difficulty in expelling the water, he should repeat Nauli several times. As a last effort to remove any lingering fluid he can use Mayurasana (the Peacock Pose).

When the student is sufficiently practised in Nauli and Aswini Mudra, so that he can open his rectum by muscular effort alone, he may dispense with the tube. Where a stream or a like body of water is not available, any sort of basin may be used, as the water rises into the colon on account of the partial vacuum that is created in doing Nauli.

Deep water is by no means necessary in order to do Basti; nor is a large quantity of water essential for the cleansing of the colon. As little as a pint can be spread throughout the colon and ejected with the contents of the bowels. Where a single flushing does not satisfactorily clear the large intestines, it may be repeated. When needed, a large quantity of buttermilk is recommended for preventing auto-intoxication. Morning is the proper time for Basti. No food should be taken prior to this flushing. This practice, it has been asserted, serves to free the body of disease, to correct the disorders of Wayu, and give the body the appearance of youth.

The value of this practice, once perfected, was quite obvious. It was clear too that once I mastered it I should never again have to suffer from constipation or any of the disorders associated with it. I should, indeed, be able to discard from my mind that such a malady existed, for my system would be under my complete control.

By now we had overstayed the time customarily set aside for visitors, so we asked for permission to leave, and I returned promptly to my room, where I began my afternoon practices.

At four o'clock I began my practices in accordance with the schedule I had set for myself. At this time I was putting the emphasis on Uddiyana and Nauli, devoting an hour to them, and doing each 1500 times.

By the end I was in a good sweat, and I thought it was high time I tried Basti. So I ordered a tub full of water. Since this was the first time that I had ever attempted to execute this practice, it was quite impossible for me to obtain any results without some mechanical aid, and I was forced to resort to the nozzle of an enema tube. By inserting this and proceeding with Nauli, I had the most astonishing experience of my life, for the intestines immediately began to fill up with water. Indeed, it was easier than taking an enema, and infinitely more successful.

This became a part of my daily discipline. Thereafter, however, I did it in the morning. With Basti, I also devoted fifteen minutes each day to Aswini Mudra, so that I might eventually dispense with the enema nozzle. I finally perfected Basti to the point where it was just as easy for me as it is for most people to take an enema.

3

It was five-thirty by the time I finished my experiment for the day, and I spent the next fifteen minutes in doing Khecari, which does not offer any physical exertion. At a quarter to six I went on my head for half an hour. I followed this with thirty minutes of Pranayama, after which I had a couple of glasses of warm milk.

This was the discipline I was to follow for the next three months, gradually increasing my head stand and breathing exercises. At the same time I was to reduce my diet, until it was to be nothing but liquids, and to diminish my sleep until it was no longer than four hours each day. The Maharishi himself never slept more than two hours a day; so I had a high standard to meet.

The only way that I could hope to maintain this rigid discipline was to take it easy, never pushing myself to the point of fatigue. It was fortunate for me that I was in excellent condition from the beginning. I had the feeling of never having been so busy in my entire life; yet here was I living in a jungle retreat, so far removed from the hurry and scurry of Western civilization. Indeed, there was not a spare minute. I had to be working constantly, never relaxing, in order to keep up.

Yet as later I looked back upon this early discipline, I often ask myself how I could have been so lazy; for after the first month I added to my regular schedule the practice of Pranayama from midnight to 1 a.m. I was forced to pick up enough sleep between my practice periods. During the last month of my training I practised at each of the four intervals of twenty-four hours. The beginner, however, is advised in no circumstances to undertake so strenuous a schedule without the constant guidance of someone thoroughly competent to judge such things. In a general way it may be said that at no time should one force oneself.

I did not try to go without sleep. I discovered, however, that it took more effort to try to sleep than it did to stay awake; so I spent the time on my practices. The same was true of my diet. At no time was I hungry. In fact, I felt as though I was eating more than was good for me, and I always stayed far within the limits of my capacity. Thus, in a sense, I took it easy.

4

On the following afternoon, during my period of relaxation, I joined my Tantrik friend and the Swamaji. They immediately inquired as to what success I had had with Basti. When I told them of my results, they were amazed. They assured me that the fact I had been able to accomplish it without any difficulty was due to the years that I had devoted to the practice of Uddiyana and Nauli before coming to India. I then asked them the meaning and purpose of the Mudras, also as to the different kinds of Mudras there were. The Swamaji undertook to answer my questions, which he did in a brief manner.

Mudra means to Seal, and Mudras consist of methods to Lock Up. Any action that serves to seal up the strength of man is a Mudra. It also means " Short," i.e., a short cut to Yoga. They are helps, and means, to various accomplishments in Yoga, being particularly useful in the early stages of breathing exercises. They give steadiness, contentment, and aid in competence. Mudras liberate men from evil influences and destroy the bonds that enslave them.

In order to awaken the sleeping Goddess (Kundalini), Mudras, accompanied by Pranayama, are practised. Mudras are substitutes for Asanas and Pranayama ; they also supplement these processes. They help to rid the body of all kinds of disease, give control over the nerves and muscles, pacify the mind, help the cleansing of the Nadis, which is the prerequisite to all Yoga practices. They likewise help the rise of the Tattwas and the awakening of the Kundalini. An important treatise of Yoga, the Gheranda Samhita, lists twenty-five of them:

1. Mhah-mudra. 2. Nabho-mudra. 3. Uddiyana. 4. Jallandhara. 5. Mulabhanda. 6. Mahabhanda. 7. Mahavedha. 8. Khecari. 9. Viparitakarani. 10. Yoni. 11. Vajroli. 12. Shaktichalani. 13. Tadagi. 14. Manduki. 15. Shambhavi. 16. Pancadharana (five dhara-

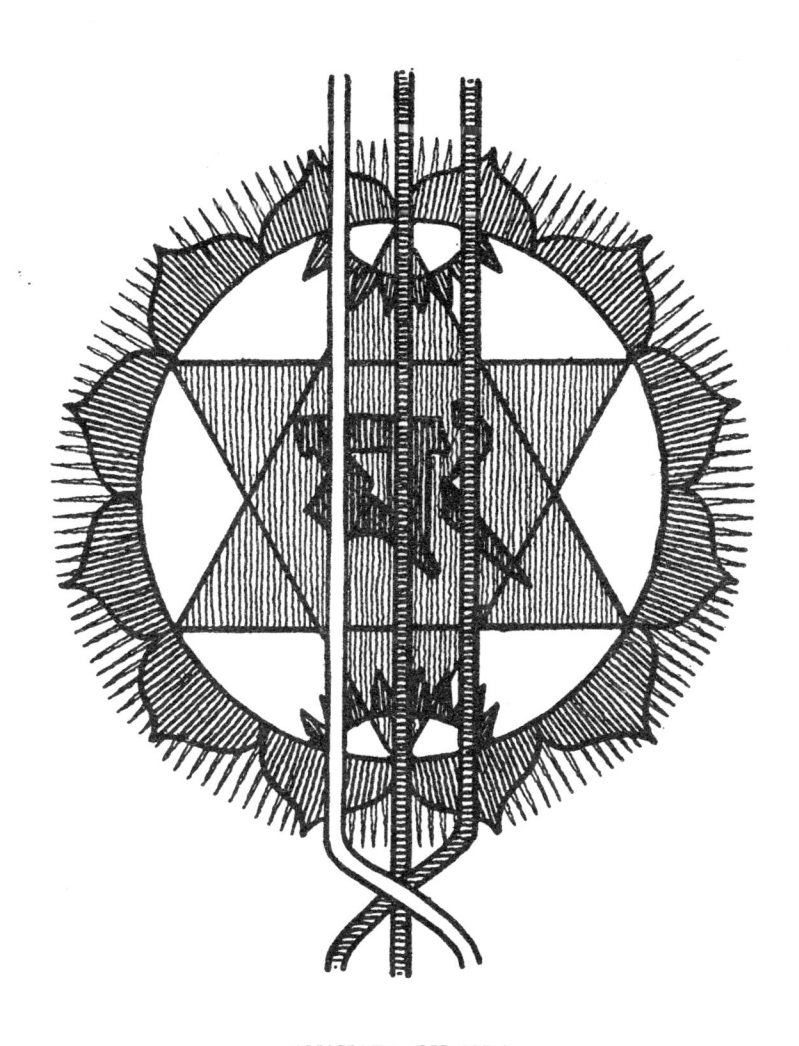

ANAHATA CHAKRA

nas.) 21. Aswini. 22. Paschini. 23. Kaki. 24. Matangi. 25. Bhujangini.

Only a few of the more important Mudras will be considered here. The student should start these practices cautiously, limiting himself to only five or ten minutes, gradually increasing the periods of practice.

5

Maha-mudra is a process of cleansing the passage to Sushumna. One takes his seat on the floor, placing the left heel at the anus, gently pressing it with the heel, then stretching forth the right leg at full length and bending forward on it, at the same time grasping the great toe of the right foot between the thumb and forefinger, the trunk coming parallel with the leg while the head is held close to the knee. In the place of the fingerhold, both hands may be locked around the ball of the foot. Then one should inhale fully through the left nostril. It is permissible to inhale through both, if necessary. One should follow this by swallowing, then stop the breath with Jalandhara-bandha and perform Uddiyana and Aswini Mudra, finally letting out the breath slowly through the right nostril.

During Kumbhaka, the eyes are to be closed and the gaze focused between the eyebrows at the root of the nose, while the mind is centred on Kundalini, upon which one should meditate as an energy resembling fire, and the bestower of whatever is desired. After practice on one side, the legs may be transposed so as to accomplish an equal number of Kumbhakas on each side. Apana, being made to move upward, enters the fire zone, and unites with Samana in the region of the navel. This flame, being struck by the air, is thereby lengthened.

Kundalini, which has been sleeping all the while and insufficiently disturbed, becomes heated in the process, and awakens. Feeling suffocated by this treatment, it rises to enter the several Chakras. The practice should be maintained for at least six months, or until Wayu enters Sushumna.

By this process the impurities of the 72,000 Nadis are washed away, and they become fit for their function; all vessels are aroused and stirred into activity. The gastric fire is increased. Even bodily decay is checked, and the one who practises the exercise will attain a faultless beauty. The exercise, when perfected, tends to destroy the deadliest poisons. Length of life is increased, the senses are conquered, the passions become wholly passive, and all sins are driven out of the mind.

This Mudra may be done solely for health purposes with no thought to awaken Kundalini. Then it will be a splendid aid in the treatment of consumption, enlargement of the spleen, difficulties due to obstructions in the bowels, colic, and diseases arising from indigestion or fever.

Inhale through the left nostril and suspend as long as possible. Then exhale through the right nostril and again suspend (external Kumbhaka) as much as you can. Start again inhaling through the left nostril. Continue the practice until the breath comes under control.

When the practice is accomplished no regulation of diet need be observed. Using the same posture, one may add Khecari Mudra, Jalandhara-bandha, and Aswini Mudra on each Kumbhaka, both on the internal and external suspensions.

Nabho Mudra consists in always keeping the tongue in the nasal cavity and restraining the breath in so far as it is possible. It should also be practised with the eyes fixed in space in a clear sky. The mind must be made blank while doing Kumbhaka.

6

Jalandhara-bandha is known as the chin lock. After swallowing, which helps to contract the muscles of the throat, the tension is kept by pressing the chin tightly against the chest, into the jugular notch as far as possible

It exercises an upward pull on the spine and spinal cord, which in turn works on the brain. The word "Jala" refers to the brain and to the nerve passing through the neck. "Dhara" denotes the upward pull.

By firmly stopping the two Nadis of the throat Prana is checked in its flow to the sixteen vital parts:

1. Thumbs. 2. Ankles. 3. Knees. 4. Thighs. 5. Prepuce. 6. Organs of generation. 7. Navel. 8. Heart. 9. Neck. 10. Throat. 11. Palate. 12. Nose. 13. The middle of the eyebrows. 14. Forehead. 15. Head. 16. Brahma Randhara.

Mulabandha is anal contraction. This is one of the principal restraints in the practice of Pranayama. By it the student is able to draw up Apana Wayu, especially necessary when trying to awaken Kundalini. It also increases the Agni in the body. Forcibly contract the anal sphincters while the perineum is closely pressed with the heel as in Siddhasana. (It may be practised with or independent of Siddhasana.) Press the left heel well against the perineum (between the anus and organs of sex) and place the right heel over the organ of generation. The abdominal wall is then carefully pressed back against the spine, as far as possible, and the anus powerfully contracted, drawing the air up by force until it goes upward to be united with Prana Wayu.

Mahabandha is the simultaneous contraction of the anus and navel. It is one of the important restraints done in Maha-mudra. It is accomplished by taking one's seat on the floor with the legs outstretched, then drawing in the left foot and placing its heel at the anus. The right foot is placed upon the left thigh. Now work the muscles of the rectum slowly but forcibly, contracting the anal sphincters of which there are two, one internal and one external, and carefully pressing in the abdominal viscera towards the spine (contracting the whole pelvic region). Then draw the Apana Wayu upward and unite it with Samana Wayu in the navel. Here again, the chin is placed in the jugular notch or the tongue lock is done. The anus thus being drawn up again and again, in time air is sure to be drawn in it, when Apana, which naturally flows downward, is forced to rise upward, thus joining Prana and Apana with Samana Wayu, which are retained in the navel. By this process all the fluids of the body are propelled toward the head. The mind is to be centred between the eyes.

After inhaling very slowly through the left nostril, swallow the breath, do Jalandhara, and follow with Kumbhaka. Now force the Prana Wayu downward, unite it with Samana Wayu, and exhale slowly through the right nostril. Start the next round with the nostril from which you last exhaled.

This exercise should be practised an equal number of times with each foot upon the thigh and always with due care. The contracting of the anal sphincters works upon the central and sympathetic nervous systems through the nerve terminals in the anal sphincters.

Prana, Apana, and Bindu (seminal fluid) are united in this active practice, giving success to the Yogi. The body is invigorated, the bones strengthened, the heart is filled with cheer, and the fear of death is removed.

While performing Mahabandha, if the Yogi fills the viscera (bowels) with air, having united Prana-Apana, then slowly directs it toward the nates, it is the process of piercing the first knot, Muladhara. This particular practice is called Mahavedha. If it is perfected, one becomes a Wayu Siddhi, that is to say, he can control the winds.

Mulabandha and Mahabandha become fruitless unless they are followed by this Mahavedha. These three must always be practised together and always with extreme caution. They confer Spiritual Powers.

7

Yoni-mudra destroys all mortal and venial sins. With a strong inspiration, fix the mind in Muladhara; then engage in contracting the generative organ. This Mudra is practised for the purpose of the study of the Tattwas. The ears are to be closed with the thumbs, the eyes with the first finger of each hand, the nostrils with the second finger, the upper lip with the third finger and the lower with the little finger of each hand. Kumbhaka is done and the mind is placed on the flame of Kundalini. The Tattwas or the lights will then arise so that one can see which is flowing by its colour and shape. This science of the Tattwas is a special one in the art of Yoga. It reveals everything that pertains to man. This Mudra is practised only when the power of Seeing has come and for the purpose of deceiving Time.

Yoga-mudra is especially useful in liberating the Serpent Power, which is technically called Kundalini. To accomplish this, first take the Padmasana Posture. The heels should press against the portion of the abdomen which they touch, the right heel exerting pressure on the pelvic loop and the left heel pressing against the cecum. The hands are now folded behind the back, the right hand grasping the left wrist. Extend these downward along the spine, exerting considerable effort. In the next step, the student bends forward and tries to lie flat upon his heels, touching the floor with his forehead. Never jerk or make any quick motion. Bend only as far as you can smoothly and comfortably. Maintain this bent position for some time.

As practice continues, the student will find himself able to make a greater bend, and in time even the last position will be found quite easy to perform. This is a splendid pelvic exercise. It builds up a powerful abdominal wall. The lumbar-sacral vertebræ receive a steady pull posteriorly and the nerves of this region are toned up. The practice tends to reduce constipation by stimulating the action of the cecum and pelvic loop and replacing the abdominal viscera. It is also found useful in overcoming seminal weakness.

The body should be held in this position from five to ten seconds. Repeat the exercise seven to ten times at a sitting. The respiration is allowed to flow as usual,

About Mudras

unless it is used to act upon Kundalini, when special Pranayama is done.

Manduka-mudra is known as the frog Mudra. You close your mouth and place the tip of the tongue at the root of the palate. There will be found a place where a ticklish sensation results. This is the place to be massaged rapidly with the tongue. After a time there will be a pleasant taste, and a quantity of saliva will flow. This is to be swallowed.

This practice checks sickness and old age. It prevents the hair from turning grey.

Shambhavi-mudra is the practice of fixing the eyes on the forehead between the eyebrows or in space.

In Yoga practices there is a great deal of internal massage. In the breathing exercises the expanding and contracting of the lungs gives a sort of massage to the heart. Abdominal exercises massage all the organs of the abdominal region and likewise for the various practices, each massaging certain organs.

8

Vajroli Mudra derives its name from the nadi which ends at the hollow of the sex organs at the neck of the bladder where it is joined by the urethra. The perfection of this Mudra gives complete control over sex.

For the perfection of the body, one should be able to control sex for one month without the slightest erection, as the loss of the vital fluid entails the loss of all the constituents of the body. It undermines the constitution and hastens the collapse of the body. A man who is weak in this respect becomes irritable on small provocation. He loses balance of mind; he becomes a slave to anger, jealousy, laziness, fear and the like. Poor memory, impotence, weak eyes, pale and bloodless face, and premature old age will overcome such men early in life.

Mind, Prana, and Semen are the three links of one chain; each supporting the other. They are the three supports to our very life. If anyone is missing or weak, to that extent the others suffer. The control of one automatically controls the others. Seminal fluid is potential power. When preserved it is indirectly metamorphosed into a subtle form called Ojuh and stored in the brain as so much mental energy, to nourish the nervous system and to be formed into Spiritual Life.

Ojuh is the finest and ultimate secretion. It is the quintessence of quintessences. It is Ojuh which keeps life going. It pervades the entire organism, enabling each organ to perform its specific function. It influences both mental and physical action. The muscles of the heart are chiefly associated with this substance, therefore the heart is considered its seat. Health and strength are latent in it. When deficient there is a diminution of bodily and mental activity; life cannot go on. Its importance cannot be over-estimated.

It is Ojuh which is mostly wasted in phthisis, anger, unhappiness, worry, excess labour, hunger, and the sex act. Ojuh is a product of the semen, consequently, when the semen is wasted, Ojuh is decreased. Upon this reciprocal relationship of Semen and Ojuh are based particular practices of Yoga.

If Bindu (seminal fluid) becomes calm and fixed, Prana Wayu becomes calm and fixed. Those who cannot practice the Mudras which pacify Bindu can take up Pranayama which gives control over Prana, and Prana will control Bindu.

The perfection of Vajroli is reached when the semen can be drawn back after it has been expelled.

Since it is impossible to give the practices of Vajroli in a book for popular publication, I will instead relate here another practice for gaining control over sex which my teacher imparted to me.

Take Siddhasana posture, inhale to your capacity through the nostril which is running at the time, then close the nostril and do Kumbhaka. Now contract the rectum and hold it contracted while the navel is contracted and expanded to its very limits. This must be done very slowly. On no occasion should the breath be held beyond an easy limit, nor should pressure be

About Mudras

exerted in any part of the practice apart from that constant grip on the rectal muscles. Before the limit of one's power of suspension is reached exhale the breath slowly through the opposite nostril.

Practise this three times at one sitting during the first month; during the second month increase to five times. By the third month an increase to ten times may be made; and to fifteen in the fourth. After this, the practice should be continued until one is able to hold the rectal muscles contracted in spite of the working of the abdominal muscles. You will, when this practice is perfected, be able to keep the anus contracted during coition. This retentive power will go on increasing with continued practice. One year's practice should give control for twenty years. This practice should, however, be kept up until the individual has obtained control over the involuntary muscles of sex so as to control semen, even if it should take longer.

The above standards are for the average man. A strong man may increase the practice to suit his capacity, but at no time should he push it to the point of strain. It is not necessary.

Those who are strong and determined may practise morning, evening, and midnight. A practice of five times daily for three months will give complete control over sex. If any pain should develop a little massage will relieve it. On no account should one miss a practice during a single day of the first three months. This is important, for Wayu will rebel and cause misery. Sexual intercourse should not be had more than twice a month until the practice is perfected. The usual diet for practising Yoga should be observed and there should be no day sleeping.

The practice of Vajroli has been a secret carefully guarded and revealed only to those who may obtain it personally from some qualified Guru. It is a practice designed especially for those who have a strong sex nature and find it extremely difficult to banish sexual desires from their minds. It is deemed unwise to include it here because there is considerable danger in trying to accomplish it without the personal guidance of one who has mastered its technique. All that I could hope to do by describing it here would be to satisfy vulgar curiosity. I say this because one must first perfect the practice of Uddiyana, Nauli, and Aswini Mudra and there is little likelihood that any among my readers will be prepared for it. Once these other practices are perfected, there will be opportunity found for them to learn this technique.

9

My time for visiting was up. I begged leave to return to my discipline. Nowhere else in the world would I have been able to break the conversation and ask my friends to excuse me in order that I might stand on my head for a while. Here it seemed natural. This is one of the reasons greater headway with these practices is made in the East. In India and other places in the East the student is surrounded with sympathetic understanding. The true significance of these apparently time-consuming and worthless exercises is appreciated. And any student who adheres to these rigid rules is looked upon with considerable respect.

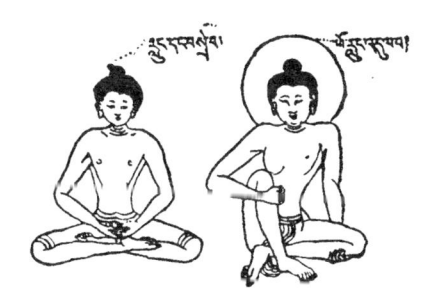

CHAPTER XVIII

MYSTIC AND ETERNAL ASPECTS OF YOGA

I

ONCE having commenced my routine, I never let down for an instant. In fact, I was continually increasing the discipline. Plans were made for the Maharishi to initiate me before my friends returned to the city. While they remained I spent every afternoon with them, plying them with questions. Often they clarified a point for me by a simple statement or example, where, otherwise, it would have required hours of reading.

I questioned them about the method of mental training as taught by Yoga, for I felt that I would advance more rapidly if I could follow their method for growth and development. Having heard of various exercises for mind control, I questioned the Swamaji and my Tantrik friend.

The training for the discipline of the mind is known as Dhyana. In order to gain mastery over Self, the student should, first of all, sit in an Asana, firmly and without movement, avoiding disturbances of light and sound and changes of temperature. Control over the body-consciousness must come first.

In the beginning this course must be exacting and rigid. The tongue should be doubled back upon itself and placed in the cavity behind the uvula, while the body remains erect and the head leans slightly forward. The eyelids should be closed but not firmly, while the eyes are directed to a point between the eyebrows. The eyeball must remain in this position, without movement. The mind must be kept free from all intruding thoughts. The breath will then become gradually steady and the steadiness of the mind will follow. Practise night and morning.

Those who tranquilize their minds can achieve perfection in the acquisition of occult powers (Siddhi). It is a saying among Buddhists that whoever commences by reflecting upon the operation of breathing and goes on through the various stages of meditation with his mind well composed will reach perfection.

Since all life comes under certain times, motions, and cycles, we find that in practising concentration it is far more favourable to adjust our practice with certain periods in the movement of the natural forces of Nature. The best period for mental activity is between midnight and sunrise. The morning between four and six is a particularly favourable time for intense concentration. The mind and body then have had their full share of rest and all nature is calm and Self-unfoldment is best obtained.

The evening is less favourable to mental activity. The lull in action and the quality of darkness tend to suspend mental action, so this period is more favourable to review meditation. Do not try to study at this time; the mind will not follow or retain what is read. From 8 a.m. to 4 p.m. the vibrations slow down to material things and from 4 p.m. to midnight they are even slower.

It must be remembered that the mind can work only between certain limits of temperature. Just as the eyes, which register light and colour only within certain limits, and the ears, which record sound only within certain limits, so does the mind have its limit of function. For the greatest mental efficiency and activity the temperature should be around 78 degrees F. For the greatest bodily efficiency at 68 degrees F.

The mind cannot work when the stomach is filled with food, nor when the blood stream is surcharged with ingested food essence. Food makes the breath vigorous

Mystic and Eternal Aspects of Yoga

and the mind, in turn, restless. Two meals a day is the best plan in the beginning. Nothing but water or a small quantity of milk should be taken between these meals.

Practice should never be overdone. Fatigue, dullness, and " mental indigestion " prevent true progress; hence moderation must be observed in habit and practice. A comfortable and steady pose should be maintained to eliminate physical disturbances and leave the mind free for efforts of concentration.

The mind may be concentrated on a light or an object of any sort. It is easier to concentrate the mind on some image, as it has a natural tendency to visualize. When one tries to project a thought it is natural to form imagines in the mind. A small disc of the moon, the size of the finger nail, with hair lines drawn on it, may be visualized, or one may take note of the respiration and fix his mind on that point of contact it makes in the head.

It is taught that six twenty-fifths of a second is the time required for a thought to pass before the consciousness. By imposing a thought upon itself and holding it before the consciousness for a period of twelve twenty-fifths of a second the thought is fixed in the mind. Deep meditation takes from one to one and one-half minutes.

Meditation is a subjective practice for fixing the thinking principle (Chitta). It brings out the first stage in liberation from action, the power to discriminate, the power to differentiate. It can be obtained only by a severe mental training which consists of identifying oneself consciously and voluntarily with something or a state of being. One must be aware of the object of meditation. He must be aware of the unity of thought which is operative, as well as the various stages of consciousness through which he passes. To combine these different features requires a singleness of mind.

2

There are three factors in the process of meditation:
1. The meditator. 2. The object of meditation. 3. The

process itself. First, the process is gradually eliminated; for with each repetition of brain action, consciousness of it diminishes, until finally it is lost altogether. That is to say, there occurs an ever-increasing ease, until in the end it comes to be performed quite automatically, quite unconsciously. Following this, the meditator is lost sight of, i.e., he is no longer conscious of himself, the mind entering the object of meditation and dwelling in its sphere. Then the mind becomes completely permeated by its association with the object. This is a state of ideation only, a state in which a thing exists potentially. After this, there follows the entire disappearance of the object, entire elimination of separateness; there is no longer any separate self, because the knower, the known, and the knowledge are one, and all truth related to it is known. There must be no play of the mind, but this does not indicate a state of inertia or forgetfulness, but a state of absolute consciousness that baffles all description. When deep reflection sets in, the objective consciousness is closed; it is then that investigation and abstract reasoning take place.

The rewards of meditation are confidence, zeal, joy, delight, and comfort. It matures the mind, puts one's heart at ease, and confers power and long life. Pride, lust, ill-will, doubt, discontent, and fear are banished, as are also dullness, sloth, and like faults. It reveals the transitory nature of all compounded things, puts an end to rebirth, and secures for one all the benefits of renunciation (non-attachment).

There are three kinds of contemplation: Gross, Subtle, and Luminous. The first is that contemplation wherein some figure, thing, or person is contemplated for qualities and attributes. The second is done on a light, such as a candle or image in the sky (mental body). The third is performed on a point of light that is evolved within the individual, or his Kundalini force.

The four themes of meditation are: 1. Impurities of the body. 2. Evils arising from sensation. 3. Ideas, or the impermanence of existence. 4. Reason and charac-

Mystic and Eternal Aspects of Yoga

ter, permanence of the Universal Law (Dharma), which is the natural condition of things or beings, the law of their existence, truth, ethical code, and the whole body of religious doctrine.

By constant systematized meditation, the mind changes its nature, gradually passing into a higher state of consciousness. In this process, every instant of elation (Ananda) is a step towards the absorption of the mind; it is a fixation of the mind on, or in, the object of its attention. By the gradual elimination of certain factors of consciousness, such as the vanity of wealth, the pomp of power, the pride of knowledge and superiority of caste or blood, this world of varieties imperceptibly passes from the mind, and one becomes rapt in concentration of the Glorious Great and Infinite.

The phases of Meditation are: 1. That in which there yet remains an awareness of the differentiation of concrete things, discursive things. 2. Enjoyment and comprehension of Universal Ideation. 3. Realization of Individual Being, apart from such Universal Ideation. The first state is one with seed, that is having some object before the mind's eye. Meditation without seed is in the complete cessation of all movement; only the essence remains. Through concentration one rises above body consciousness, through meditation one rises above the mind.

3

Preparation for meditation consists in bringing the mind into perfect stillness. The practice of concentration should never be attempted when the breath is disturbed. Meditation should not be practised in the daytime, when Pingala (right breath) is flowing; nor at night, when Ida (left breath) is flowing. Complete silence is essential during meditation. There must be no duality, no sleep, no wakefulness, no remembering, no forgetting.

It is an elementary form of meditation when the student, after taking his posture, closes his eyes and causes his breath to flow smoothly and easily and then draws upon his imagination to create a beautiful situation which is the symbol of his highest ideals. It should represent to him some spiritual concept: Christ, the Virgin Mary, Buddha, Krishna, or some other deity, or the face of his Guru. This he puts in his heart, where he surrounds the image with an ocean of light, or nectar, and holds it while mentally reviewing his creations. Any sort of beautiful situation may be created. It will differ according to one's imaginative capacity. When built up, this concept and this alone must be constantly meditated upon. Do not change from one to another. First master one and perfect it. Only then will the feelings be sufficiently assured to allow another, if one so chooses.

At first it will be found that the mind can be held for only a few moments on the chosen imagery. When it wanders it must be brought back again and again to the same concept. Meditation must continue, and gradually it will respond to the student's commands. Zealous, ardent, strenuous, and continuous effort will bring perception of Aura and visions of Forms. When these Forms come, they must not be contemplated too closely, else they will disappear.

One should endeavour to bring meditation to a duration of three hours, or even more, if it be possible.

A well-trained mind can be fixed at will on any object to the exclusion of all else. The waves in the mind stuff are stilled and a perfected condition set up to reflect the truth that is within.

In order that I might check myself, the Swamaji related a few simple practices to me. One simple aid to meditation is a candle. Place a lighted candle on a table, level with the eyes, or slightly lower, and some eighteen inches from the eyes. Rest the elbows on the table and hold the eyelids open with the thumb and forefinger of each hand. Look into the flame of the candle for five or more minutes, or until the tears begin to flow. Do not rub the eyes as this water is impure.

Next close the eyes, making a cup-like shape of the

palms and place them over the eyes. One should now see a mental image of the candle flame, very small in size. One must control this image, keeping it before the mental vision as long as possible. Try to keep it stationary or move it only with your own will.

On the physical side this practice strengthens the eyes, making them bright and attractive. The solar plexus is acted upon and the student will find that charm is added to the personality. On the mental side, this practice is held in high regard as a practice in concentration.

Concentration on the light in the middle of the forehead between the eyes after having done the candle exercise is called subtle contemplation. One may also contemplate on an ocean of light in the heart or on a flame in the region of the navel. The body has lights of different quality which, with practice, may be seen and understood. The lights of the Tattwas are dull, while mental lights are bright. Ojuh light is seen while one is still conscious. When the highest light is manifest there is no sense consciousness.

Concentration may be done on these lights. A time will then come when you can bring this light into the mental space at will and thereby develop a powerful intention.

One of the purification processes is really a practice in concentration. It is known as Trataka. One looks steadily at some small object, without blinking, holding the eyelids slightly more open than usual, and continues until the eyes water. Then close the eyes and roll the eyeballs a few times. Rinse carefully with cold water. The purpose of this practice is to co-ordinate the motor and sensory nerves. This helps to produce the state of calm essential to concentration. Trataka preserves a clear eyesight and gives immunity from diseases of the eye.

The tensing and relaxing method of concentration is accomplished by making an effort to crop the appearance of each thought instantly it arises. Keep a steady watch for each thought in its formation and stop it immediately. At the beginning this will tax the mind considerably. When the mind becomes tense and control is lost, let it wander for a while. Relax completely and observe its fancies, its gambols, while it roams here and there. Do this until fully rested, then try to take hold of it again. Cut off each idea at the instant it comes up. As the practice improves, the stream of ideas instead of being cut short will seem to rise with increasing rapidity. This is an indication that the student is making headway, that his mind is becoming clearer, his observation sharper. This is the real state of the mind's operation. From this point, the mind is to be perfectly relaxed. Watch it as an onlooker, allowing it full sway to the end that it will of itself slow down and each operation may be studied minutely to the ultimate result of its complete movement being brought under control. When its absolute suspension can be reached for a period of time such as it takes to puncture a lotus leaf with a needle, then higher processes of Yoga become necessary. This moment of positive suspension is sufficient to make the Yogi realize his Real Self. A tranquil state is reached when the thoughts seem to arise so fast they cannot be counted.

Various sounds may be heard in the ears. They are only the motion of Prana in the Nadis. No anxiety should be felt. One may use them for the fixation of the mind. In time, as the mind becomes absorbed in meditation, they will pass away.

Visions of whatever sort are but the creation of one's own mind and have no extraneous existence whatsoever. These may also be used for concentration. They should never cause the slightest anxiety.

4

Another excellent method of concentration is known as **Chhaya Pursha Sadhana** or Cultivation of the Shadow Man.

Take a position in the sun when the sky overhead is perfectly clear and your shadow falls directly in

Mystic and Eternal Aspects of Yoga

front of you for about your own length. Centre your attention on your shadow at the point of the shoulders and base of the neck. Hold this view with the eyes steady, the lids slightly dilated, for as long as you can. When the eyes become tired and begin to water freely, close and open them a few times, raise the head and gaze into space toward the clear sky where you will see a figure, a full grey shadow, capable of appearing in many colours. Hold this figure in concentration as long as you possibly can. By regular practice the time will come when the shadow will be transparent. Eventually you will see features on the shadow, and finally these features will turn and face you and you will be looking at yourself. This is concentration. It may be used in the usual practice of Yoga. Practice may be done under the moon in those localities where the moon sheds its rays in splendour. With a practiced Yogi this invoking of the shadow man may be used to determine whether the time is auspicious for important affairs. The character of the shadow will reveal matters of one's own fate, even foretelling death. It reveals the state of the Tattwas in one's body, which in turn reveals all things.

It is said that if the practice is done for twelve years, the shadow will be with one both day and night, giving guidance insight into one's future. This practice is suited to those localities only where cloudless skies are to be found over several months.

In kind, this practice is just as important as the candle. After a long time this shadow can be made to appear to one, rising and leaving the body through the portal of the eyes. Eventually this can be projected on a screen or wall. It is subtle and very changeable, because the apparition is mixed with the air in the vacuum of the sky. When the Yogi can perceive every part of his form in the reflected shadow he obtains perfect control over breath, and good results from every act. By seeing his mental body he will know all things about himself. When this state is reached, passions become completely passive and salvation is attained.

5

Still another practice is known as Sukshma Dhyana or Luminous Contemplation. This is done by fixing the gaze in space, without blinking. Practising on one's image by the shadow method is also Luminous Contemplation. These practices once perfected, the Yogi attains the power of placing any sort of picture upon a dark screen to learn what he desires to know. By these practices, there comes a time when there is direct perception of Self. The Yogi also attains the power to see Kundalini, which otherwise cannot be seen on account of its subtleness and great changeability. This, however, can occur only after it is awakened.

In Kundalini is the Jiva (Soul) with the form of a candle flame. This may be used for contemplation. In the Navel is the centre of the Sun Light connected with the element of Fire. When contemplating this, it is Fire Meditation. If the student always thinks of this light, until it becomes a part of his daily life and he feels he is walking in it, he will be able to realize Siddhis, or powers of a rare kind and value.

Exhale all air, draw in the solar plexus (Uddiyana) and practise meditation on the heart centre. This will awaken the light therein and transmute sex energy.

In order to contemplate upon the void it is necessary to do what is known as Unmani Mudra (no mind). Keep the attention fixed upon as insipid an idea as possible or make the mind blank. There will result an outgoing of ideas and will. With repetition this can be done quite automatically. The object is to become void inside and out. You can put Prana wherever you desire in your body by thinking of yourself as hollow inside and sending your thought current wherever you want it to go. When all thoughts are banished, the mind loses its identity, as salt disappears in water. One will be amply rewarded, long before this stage is fully reached, by the attainment of Siddhi, such as clairvoyance.

Shambhava Mudra effects the absorption of the mind

and brings happiness. It is accomplished by staring into space without seeing anything. Simply gaze fixedly ahead without blinking the eyelids, the lids slightly dilated. Adopt a stony stare. Contemplate space by rendering the mind void of all thought. The mind must be in a state of complete emptiness. Let no external thing make any impression on the retina of the eye, though they remain wide open.

This practice will bring the breath under control, correct nervous conditions, enable the student to overcome troublesome moods, remedy an undesirable mental state, destroy self-consciousness, and permit him to know what is happening around him. By giving the mind this monotonous tone, which is like a vacuum, it will attain magnet-like qualities. The internal world will rush in from the subjective side. This practice places the mind in a state of watchful waiting, and Truth becomes its normal companion.

There is another method of attaining Unmani (no mind) which is known as Nasagra Drishti (Nasal Gaze). Fix the gaze on the tip of the nose with the eyebrows slightly raised, and the mind contemplating the light (Life Energy) in the heart. One must think of this Life Energy inwardly, while apparently looking outward. This is a splendid exercise for the wandering mind and should be practised over a period of several months.

An important practice in meditative poses is the Frontal Gaze. This is a splendid exercise for the unsteady mind and useful to the accomplishment of Unmani. Fix the eyes upon a spot between the eyebrows, the lids closed loosely and allowing them to find their own restful place which will leave them slightly open with the whites of the eyes visible. This frontal gaze is practised as a part of Siddhasana, or independently of it. Like the nasal gaze, it must be done with caution, especially if the nerves are easily excited.

The eyelids are to remain slightly open in both these instances. Roll back the eyes and concentrate upon the forehead. You can then perceive the lustre from the Great Soul and your worldly feelings will be annihilated or absorbed into the soul.

Suppress the keen desire to open the eyes for an instant and look about. This is the desire of the physical body, seeking as ever to express itself and to escape the commands put upon it.

The student who can contemplate the void, or space, while walking or standing or dreaming, becomes absorbed in the ether. To realize this state is to attain the unconditional or " Divine Body of Truth." A Yogi, desiring success, should acquire the power of habitual practice. It produces wonderful effects, the feeling is indescribable. You become a changed man, purged from sin and hindrances of all kinds. You live a new life and become universally beloved. You acquire psychic powers.

This is one of the processes of emancipation. By making the mind functionless, one becomes saturated with Sattwaguna.

6

The form of Yoga which deals with the absorption of the mind in sound is known as Laya Yoga. It consists in losing oneself in some internal object and seeking to hear mystic sounds.

This practice is done by sitting in Siddhasana, with eyes fixed on the spot between the eyebrows, the eyeballs turned upward so that the lids remain half closed. The eyes, ears, nose, and mouth are to be shut off with the fingers. Then listen with a collected mind for a sound in the right ear. Eventually a clear sound will be heard. In the beginning the sounds are very loud and of great variety, but with increasing practice they become more and more subtle. At first they surge like the beating of a kettle drum ; in the intermediate stages they are more like the sounds produced by a conch shell ; in the last stage they resemble the sound of a flute or of bees. All these sounds are reproduced in the body and cannot be heard by anyone else. One should practise with both the loud and subtle sounds, going from one to the other, since in this manner the distracted mind will not be inclined to wander elsewhere.

When the Yogi's mind is attentively engaged in this sound, he becomes ensnared by it and distractions are overcome. The mind gives up all its activities and becomes calm, craving no enjoyment, and becomes one with the breath. Trance is induced, when the Yogi forgets all external things, losing consciousness of himself. When the mind is absorbed in itself, he attains cosmic consciousness, eternal bliss. Those who have experienced drowning will understand this.

This absorption produced by the mind entering Nada (sound) immediately gives spiritual powers, with a sort of ecstasy. One forgets all his material existence. This absorption is called Moksha (Liberation). What is heard in the form of sound is Shakti power, that which is formless, the first stage of the Tattwas. Tattwa is the "seed." Hatha Yoga is the "field," and indifference the "water." By the action of these three the Yogi abolishes the mind and advances understanding.

Desiring the Kingdom of Yoga one must, with the mind collected and free from all cares, take up this practice of hearing Anahata Sound (in the heart) and determine to practise it constantly. It must be heard attentively. The mind then is combined with sound and loses its own unsteadiness. At length this meditation waxes hot, and the intense mental concentration causes vital elixir to drain from the skull. This passes through the upper Nadis where it unites with Prana (mind substance) and nourishes the soul. These internal sounds of the body can be heard only by those whose Nadis are free from all impurity and practised in Pranayama.

Concentration upon the organs of the body involved in the various exercises greatly increases the sensitiveness of those parts and intensifies and strengthens them to a marvellous degree. Just as with the organs of sense, if your thoughts dwell on any part of the body, sensation rushes to that part and, to the consciousness, it momentarily appears to be the only existent part. If we dwell on this, the powers of various parts can be awakened.

Meditation upon the centre to which you feel the pressure rising after a complete Kumbhaka (suspension) gives access to the light of Ojuh. Focus this light where you will. The first time it is seen in a flash or in constant motion; then, as you mount to the sense plane, it will become increasingly illuminating. One important purpose in Yoga is to obtain this light.

Concentration shows itself in five progressive mental stages: Analysis, Reflection, Fondness, Bliss, and Concentration. The student in the first stage gains knowledge of the nature of Form and arrives at ordinary concentration. The second step is one of reflection alone. Here the lower stage of analysis is transcended. In the third, reflection gives way to a blissful state of consciousness and later, in the fourth stage, this merges into pure ecstacy. In the fifth stage, sensation, though always apparent, becomes suppressed and gives way to complete concentration, a state of " mere existence." In Samadhi there is neither seeing nor hearing, neither physical nor mental consciousness, only pure existence.

When practising meditation, one sees the mark on closing his eyes or on entering into his chamber or any other place; it is called the Acquired Mark. When he meditates by making this mark his artifice, he sees a light. From this state on, not taking any notice of the mark, he concentrates his thoughts on that light which emanates from the mark. By long and assiduous practice he is able to spread this light over the entire Universe.

7

It would take me a long time to fully digest and to comprehend everything which my teacher related to me that afternoon. I did not waste any time, however, in making notes on it. During the following days, before

Mystic and Eternal Aspects of Yoga

my Tantrik friend and the Swamaji returned to the city, I questioned them again on those points which I found missing when I tried to write up my notes. Not only was I going to follow the physical practices of Hatha Yoga but I was going to adhere to their form of mental discipline.

As I developed my Pranayama, it was necessary to understand fully the function of the mind and how to gain the fullest control over it. That very afternoon I began to observe the mind in its rambles and analyse all its activities. I took notes, so I could see the development I was making as a result of the practices. I soon discovered how undeveloped my mind was at this stage and realized that it would be some time before I could benefit by the practice of Trataka or produce the Shadow Man.

Adhering to this rigid discipline, the days flew by like minutes. Never had I been so occupied, for I had not one second to spare. At the end of the second week, the Maharishi initiated me. This was a simple initiation for the purpose of establishing a conscious tie between us. Thus he would know what inner progress I was making. This also enabled him to help me over many obstacles which I encountered during my meditations and reflections. The initiation was somewhat similar to the one I have already described.

After this, my Tantrik friend and the Swamaji returned to the city for a couple of months. They knew I had more than enough to keep me busy, and now it was entirely up to me. I had to arrive at another stage of growth, and this could come only through the practices which I was following.

Could I hold to this rigid discipline which they assured me would net such great results?

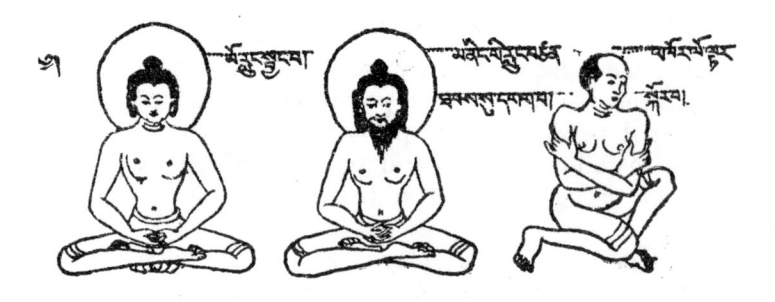

CHAPTER XIX

KUNDALINI

I

For three months I had practised my discipline before my friends returned to our Jungle Retreat. They were very eager to hear what progress I had made. In the West I would have broken my normal life to welcome visitors and celebrate their return. But here it was the camp of a Yogi, and my discipline continued as usual while my friends waited for visiting hours to see me.

In the beginning I found a few of the practices a little distressing, but I did not give up. I overcame the obstacles and brought the external aspects of the practices up to perfection. Whether I had developed my inner consciousness to the same degree remained to be discovered. They were going to instruct me in tests to enable me to find out.

I had followed their instructions and never given the goal the slightest concern. I had found my joy in the practices. I knew growth came only through activity and I considered this opportunity for discipline the greatest blessing of my life.

By the time my friends returned I had been able to reduce my diet to nothing but liquids, which seemed to be more than enough. Four hours' sleep was enough and even this had to be broken, for I had carried my discipline to the point where I practised three hours at a time four times a day. I did not feel any strain, however ; on the contrary I was as fresh as a child.

There had been little difficulty in developing the head stand to the point of doing it for an hour at a time; this I had done before I left the United States. By placing it at three intervals I was able to spend the required three hours on my head each day. There is no other practice which enables one to experience such complete relaxation. The inner consciousness floods the mind; this is its greatest advantage. With this practice comes a strong tendency toward philosophical inquiry and perception which brings joy in its wake.

If the student desires to discover the unsteady state of the mind in which he is living, there is no better way than to stand on the head and observe what takes place. You will be amazed. Try it and see.

After assuming the position, forget everything and try objectively to watch the mind. At first, you will hear sounds and find the mind racing in all directions. Let it race. Now try to follow some line of thought. You will find the mind wants to think about anything but the chosen subject. As practice is developed, however, and the body conditioned, the mind begins to subside slowly. It will not be long before the mind will come to a standstill, at which time it will be possible to attend to the chosen thought. After I developed the practice I found that all time was banished, yet some little inner mechanism kept track of its passing. I would go up on my head, bring my mind to a given point and there I would leave it. From that instant I was completely unaware of the passing of time.

My friends were anxious to know how I had been progressing with my Pranayama. At the time of their arrival I had brought my Kumbhaka up to the required time. I had had great difficulty in doing this. Various Asanas helped over a few of the early obstacles, but when I reached six minutes I found I had to increase the time of my Bhastrika. This appeared to be the normal limit for me and I experienced considerable pressure caused by the impulse to breathe again. This is where I discovered the purpose of Khecari Mudra.

By swallowing my tongue I was able to overcome this natural impulse. Then came the task of gaining control over the breath and swallowing in such a manner as to let it pass into the stomach and intestines instead of permitting it to escape. It was through this process that I was able to bring about the necessary pressure required to awake that subtle energy of the body known as Kundalini.

I had finally been able to dispense with the enema nozzle and did Basti without mechanical aid. Through the perfection of this technique as well as of Vajroli I gained complete control over the nerve centre in that region which is the seat of Kundalini.

2

I was constantly questioning my friends on Kundalini, and the theory on which it is based. I wanted to know all about its nature. They gave me a general outline of its principles and the techniques pertaining to it.

The ultimate success of all Yoga practices depends upon awakening Kundalini. On Kundalini is founded the whole of Hatha Yoga teachings and practices. The nervous system furnishes the physiological basis of this system of Yoga. Without this knowledge it is quite impossible to carry out its practices.

Hence the aim and most important achievement sought by a Sadhaka is the awakening of the Kundalini. Ordinarily this force never awakens in man unless developed by Yoga practices. It is said that so long as Kundalini is asleep in the body the Jiva (soul) is like a brute, and true knowledge will not arise, although the student practises Yoga all his life. It is only through the awakening of Kundalini that the deadening covers of matter are removed. He who moves this Shakti enters upon the path which releases one from all bondage. By our breathing we are connected with the Universal Life Principle. It is there that each particular life melts and mingles with the One Life.

Kundalini

As a power Kundalini is the highest manifestation of consciousness in the body. Kundalini represents the creative force of the world as manifest in man. It is eternally engaged in creation. Ordinary creation is from spirit to matter, but Yoga reverses this process and seeks to change matter into spirit. It is creative energy in a static state, spiritual force itself, "The Grand Potential," the residual power remaining after the creation of the world, a gross form of Prakriti (Cosmic Energy). It embodies all powers and assumes all forms; it is the seat of all bodily and mental manifestations. According to the Cosmic principle there must be a static background in any sphere of activity of energy, hence the bodily forces necessarily presuppose some static support, since a dynamic aspect can never be without its static counterpart.

In all life this is Kundalini. Pranic forces are but the motion of Kundalini, which is the static centre of the whole body. There must first be a neutral centre for the manifestation of all energy. The forces which emanate from this neutral point traverse the whole body form and return to it, just as electricity runs out the positive pole of a battery and returns to it by the negative. This central part of the body is said to be the reflected neutral centre manifestation of all forces which act from the brain in the living human frame. As magnetism is latent at the central part of a magnet so is Kundalini in the body centre.

3

Kundalini is said to be the mother of the three qualities: Sattwaguna, Rajaguna, and Tamaguna. "Sat" means existence, light, illumination. "Raj" means activity and "Tam" means darkness, the obstructing quality. They might be expressed as the qualities of construction, destruction, and regulation. This vital spot is like a root in the body. It is the static or potential body-energy, the central body-power, the fountain-head of Knowledge. From its seat this body vehicle is born, from that seat the mind is born, and from Kundalini, Agni (the Promethean Fire of Life) becomes augmented. From the seat of Kundalini rises Wayu (bodily energy), Bindu (the seed of life) and Nada (sound).

Kundalini, it must be understood, is not an object of hearing but a most subtle thing in the form of light. It is the power from which all nature's gifts proceed. Just as all the powers of this Universe exist in God, so do all the powers of each individual exist in Kundalini.

It is this Shakti which mainly lies back of the performed wonders of the Yogi. In the running Wheel of Life Kundalini may be likened to the imperceptible motion at the axle, the sweep of the periphery being respiration.

Manifest energy has three aspects: Neutral, Centripetal and Centrifugal. In the nervous system centripetal currents are called sensory or afferent currents. The centrifrugal currents are called motor or efferent currents. These currents have their neutral state in the Muladhara Chakra (Kundalini). Oxygen and nutrition are taken in by centripetal currents. Waste and effete matter are thrown out by centrifugal currents. Vital force, which is back of all manifestations of nerve force, must not be mistaken for functions of the brain or heart or any other part of the body which are created by it. One must not mistake the things created for the Creator.

The position of Kundalini is said to be at the upper border of the triangular piece of bone of the spinal column which is wedged between the two hip bones, known as the sacrum. It is about half-way between the navel and the sex organs, some nine inches above the perineum. This space is the root; from here come the seventy-two thousand Nadis. Kundalini, soft and shining, enhaloed with a mass of Golden Light, illuminating by its own Light, lies here in a lethargic state, coiled three and one-half times, covering with its face the entrance of Sushumna (Brahma Nadi). It is symbolized by a snake having three and one-half coils, with its tail in its mouth.

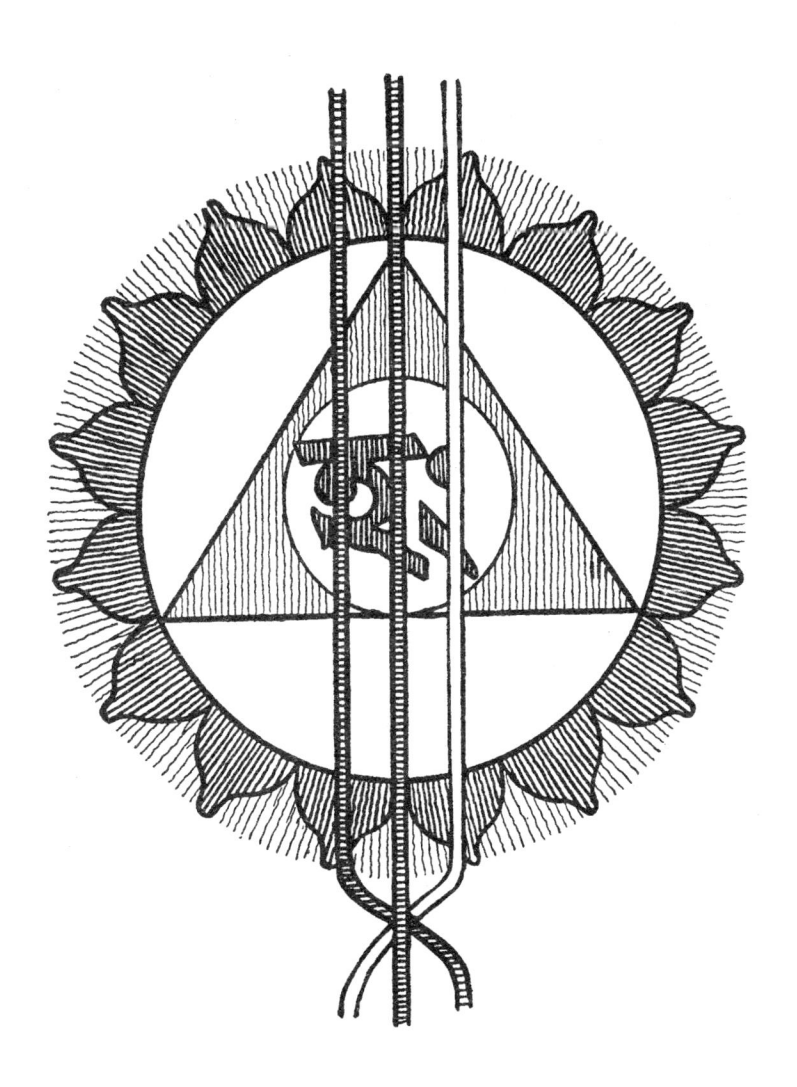

VISHUDDHA CHAKRA

The object of Yoga is to awaken the Vital Force, Kundalini, which moves in Sushumna where it ultimately reaches Brahmarandra, The Thousand-Petalled Lotus in the head. Anyone who awakens Kundalini and renounces all fruits of action attains the condition of Samadhi, and the door to Brahma is unlocked. When Kundalini is aroused, it becomes but a matter of time and practice until all the Chakras may be penetrated in successive stages. This is accomplished by means of special postures, Mudras and the practice of Kumbhaka. The perfection of the different techniques is essential, because each has its specific purpose. Jalandhara Bandha and Mula-bandha check the downward tendency of Prana. Aswini Mudra makes Apana go upward. Uddiyana Bandha makes the united Prana-Apana enter Sushumna. Through Shaktichalana one forces the Kundalini from Muladhara upward through the plexi. All of this is wellnigh impossible without the aid of a Guru.

First a strict Yoga diet must be followed and coition must be foregone for at least a month. No superconscious state is possible without awakening Kundalini. First organic action is stopped, then comes the trance or complete suspension of animation. All inner and outer forces are subdued, the mind identifies itself with its source.

Kundalini is both light and sound, and for this reason Mantra Yoga is often used to arouse it. Mantra is endowed with powers of action and sensation, and it circulates throughout the body. That almost imperceptible sound of the breath is called Mantra, designated as Hamsa. " Ham " is the outward flow, and " Sa " the inward. The Jiva (Soul) has its suppport in the Hamsa. This Mantra is uttered twenty-one thousand and six hundred times in twenty-four hours.

The terms Bija Mantra and seed Mantra, and there is a specific one connected with each Chakra, represent the energy which rests therein. By use of the seed Mantra control of the respective centres is attained.

A brief explanation of the physiological working of Mantra might make this a bit clearer. It is known that the sense organs respond to vibrations within certain limits. The limit may be extended or diminished. With constant repetition of stimulus to nervous centres, reaction is not only increased but a permanent alteration occurs. Likewise a change in the function of nervous energy is caused by the action of the breath in the practice of Mantra. The formula of Mantra is the most esoteric of all Yoga.

The Yogi, fixing his attention on the Mantra, doing it faithfully for one hundred thousand or more times, attains Siddhi. All his desires are granted. Even a person who is heavily burdened with past Karma attains success by Mantra Yoga if he but repeats his Mantra two hundred thousand times. He gains the power of attracting others, and these remain always under his control, if he raises his practice to three hundred thousand times. When he has repeated the Mantras six hundred thousand times, he becomes a vehicle of power. The practice is then raised to one million, and on to a million and a half, a million and eight hundred thousand, two million and eight hundred thousand and three million times. Each accomplishment like that of breath control gives added power and perfection.

4

A word here about Siddhis seems pertinent. They come to the disciple masked, once his Prana and mind are under control. When these begin to rise and take form, there appears before the mind a phenomenon in the form of a mist (or smoke), of hot air, of wind, of fire, of lightning, of a crystal, of the moon. These are all experiences or stages on the path to Siddhis.

Siddhis are spoken of as possessions ; they can become hindrances exposing the possessor to evil tendencies. They are not evil in themselves and become evil only when they are the instrument of demeritorious actions. They can be a wonderful stimulus to progress if kept secret and applied only on the most carefully considered occasions.

Now let me relate some of the methods for awakening Kundalini which were given me by my teacher on various occasions.

Put a soft ball or pad in such a position as to exert pressure on the space between the sex organs and the anus when in the Siddhasana or Padmasana posture. Then practise Khecari Mudra. The eyes focused rigidly between the eyebrows, Kumbhaka should be done and then Jalandhara. Now contract the anus and navel and press the breath to the lower end of Sushumna instead of permitting it to go to Ida or Pingala. The Agni will flame up, owing to the flow of Wayu. This enables Kundalini to pierce the primary Nadi, Sushumna, after which it can be made to open all Chakras. When Sushumna is opened one feels the ascent of the fire to the brain. It is as if a hot current of air were blown through a tube from the bottom to the top. The release of the power in the Chakras causes them to tremble, and the Kundalini becomes absorbed in the " Great Soul."

When the student undertakes to awaken Kundalini he should keep this Shakti constantly before his mind. He should think of it as extending to the tip of the tongue and pay obeisance to it with every bit of food and drink he takes.

Another variation of this technique is to sit on a cotton ball, made secure with a bandage, so that it will press the perineum, then extend the limbs, keeping them stiff with the feet apart. Now place the head on the knees, and grasp the great toes with the thumb and forefinger of each hand, holding the trunk as close as possible to the thighs. Inhale through the left nostril and do Kumbhaka with tension on the anus and navel. This act of pulling them together forces Prana into the Sushumna Nadi. When fatigued, exhale through the right nostril and repeat by inhaling through this same nostril. Continue for a while this breathing pro-

Kundalini

cess of alternating from one nostril to the other; however always finish the practice by exhaling through the left nostril.

5

One of the most important of the Mudras is known as Shaktichalana, which is another practice to awaken Kundalini.

Kundalini, which is asleep in the Muladhara Chakra, is energized and begins to move when it is agitated by Apana Wayu. First take the Baddha Padmasana. If unable to assume this Asana, Siddhasana may be substituted. Inhale through the right nostril, do Jalandhara and centre the eyes on the tip of the nose or between the eyebrows. Suspend in the Svadhishthana Chakra, which is the Water Centre. Then close the rectum by Aswini Mudra and draw in the navel by performing Uddiyana. Before the suspension has weakened, exhale very slowly through the left nostril. Repeat over and over again. In this way the Serpent Kundalini begins to feel suffocated and rises upward. Follow this by Yoni Mudra.

To force Kundalini into Sushumna, one must work for an hour and thirty minutes. Practise Bhastrika and then work Kundalini by performing several hundred rounds of Nauli. In the course of time it will come alive. This accomplishment will be hastened if the student lives on rice, milk sweetened with pure cane sugar, barley broth, and a few fruits.

This practice should be continued for, at least, forty minutes each day, in order to produce any results. If one can devote more time, he will be rewarded accordingly. Lack of will power will, of course, mean delay or failure. Not all individuals are qualified to practise Hatha Yoga. The root word "Hat" means determination.

The effectiveness of this practice has been demonstrated again and again; so do not despair if it takes a little more time than expected, to reach results. It is best to begin the practice with a few rounds of Bhastrika. Physical pain must be withstood.

6

Here is a short-cut method for the awakening of Kundalini which my teacher related to me.

Take a cloth of some soft material and fold it several times into a pad about nine inches square and four inches thick. Place this upon the navel and tie in position. Taking one's seat in Siddhasana, suspend and follow with Jalandhara, Uddiyana, and Aswini Mudra. The greater the pull on the rectum the better. Then practise Nauli until Kundalini is moved. If this practice is done for forty minutes each day, Kundalini should be brought to life in one year. A warning should be added cautioning the student never to carry Kumbhaka to such a point that sudden exhalation is imperative.

7

There are several forms of Kumbhaka that the pupil must know. One of them is called Bhramari Kumbhaka or the Beetle-Droning Kumbhaka. This is done in the middle of the night when there is not a sound to be heard. While the Yogi is practising his Kumbhaka he should close his ears with the hands and listen attentively for sounds in his right ear. These sounds will be heard readily through daily practice. They are of ten kinds: 1. Like the hum of a bee. 2. Like the sound from a bamboo flute. 3. Like the ringing of bells. 4. Like the sound of a conch shell. 5. Like the sound from a stringed instrument (Vina). 6. Like a silver cymbal. 7. Like a kettle drum. 8. Like a clay drum or trumpet blast. 9. Like thunder. 10. The Anahata Sound rising from the heart.

This last sound has a resonance in which there is a light where the mind should be fixed. When it becomes absorbed here, the mind reaches the seat of Vishnu, bringing positive success in Samadhi.

This practice is preparatory to Rasananda-Yoga Samadhi which begins with Bhramari Kumbhaka. After doing Bhramari slowly expel the breath, making a buzzing sound like that of a bee.

Kundalini

Another form of Kumbhaka is known as Murchchha Kumbhaka. It renders the mind passive and induces fainting. You sit in Siddhasana and then inhale through both nostrils. Then swallow, and do Jalandhara and Aswini Mudra. Now, with the pressure in the lower abdominal region, expel the air slowly. Follow this with an external Kumbhaka, which will cause the mind to swoon, producing a sense of comfort. Should fainting occur, you can be sure that Kumbhaka has been successful. To complete Murchchha, Shaktichalana must be practised along with it. This practice is especially effective in producing mental passivity.

Another important form of Kumbhaka in which my teacher instructed me was Kevala Kumbhaka. It consists in retaining the full length of breath in the body, without any physical or muscular effort, so that none of it may escape. It is said that this practice cures all diseases, promotes longevity, removes the darkness of mind, enlightens the moral nature, purges one from all sins and awakens the soul. This state is Samadhi, and the breath of the practiser becomes absorbed in the Great Soul.

The Chitta, i.e., feeling consciousness, can be perfectly directed, and the Yogi can easily attain perfection in everything he desires. To be sure, you have to be well skilled in the various practices of breathing before you can undertake this Kevala Kumbhaka, and be master of complete concentration of mind, reaching the point of trance, in which thoughts become visualized.

After perfecting Khecari Mudra and living in the regulation subterranean retreat, the Yogi reduces his diet to that of rich milk only, on which he subsists for an entire six months. He follows this by living on Ghee and milk for about a week. Then he abstains from all foods for a day or two. Now, consciously counting the number of his respirations, he doubles the normal and practises this for a time. Then he fills the lungs with air and shuts both nostrils. The glottis is pressed backward by the tip of the tongue, and the tongue is swallowed into the fascia. Thus he suspends his breath, at the same time focusing his eyes between the eyebrows, or on the tip of the nose. His mind becoming dead, he attains spiritual power.

8

The Yogi's senses are suspended when he can suspend his respiratory movements for ten minutes and forty-eight seconds. Dharana is attained when the breath can be held for twenty-one minutes and thirty-six seconds. Dhyana is attained when the breath is held for forty-three minutes and twelve seconds. Samadhi is attained when the breath is held for one hour, twenty-six minutes and twenty-four seconds. The synthesis of these final three stages of Yoga is known as Samyama.

When the Yogi has accomplished Kumbhaka to the point of holding the breath for two and a half to three hours, he has attained extraordinary powers, such as hearing sounds at great distances, seeing objects which are out of sight, covering long distances quickly, and other phenomena usually considered impossible.

The Yogi can conquer the five elements of Earth, Water, Fire, Air, and Ether when he can retain his "Breath of Life" for a period of two and a half hours in their respective centres: Muladhara, Svadhishthana, Manipura, Anahada, and Vishuddha. This gives him knowledge of these five elements, so that they no longer can deter him, and it is in his power to enjoy them constantly.

When the Yoga has learned to restrain his breath for three hours, he is able to combine his soul with the "Great Soul." During this stage no thoughts will cross his mind, even for a moment. His passions become completely passive, and he passes without effort to the Divine and Universal. He can support himself on a single finger, and even travel in space like a cotton-tree seed. When he has succeeded in restraining his breath for three hours, he need practise Pranayama but once daily.

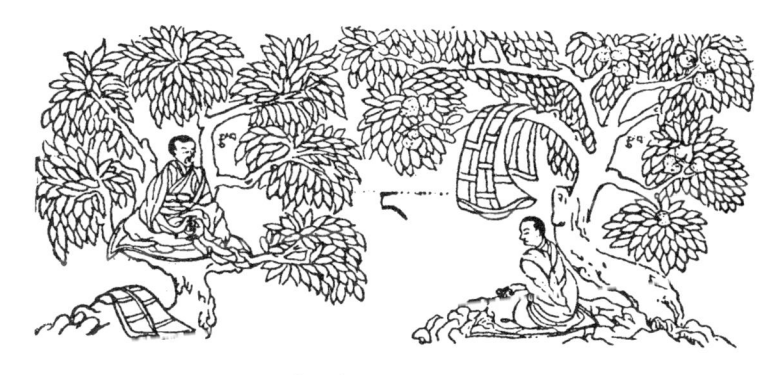

CHAPTER XX

MY FINAL INITIATION

I

FOR the next few days I was told to direct all my discipline toward a supreme effort to awaken Kundalini and become consciously aware of it. The Maharishi had started the preparations for my ultimate Initiation which was for the purpose of awakening Kundalini. But, as it had been so often pointed out to me, this supreme experience could be mine only through my own effort. All that my teachers and the Maharishi could do for me was to guide me along the path. During the next few days and I did not waste an instant. I spared no energy. I gave all of myself to the final effort.

The tests were given me. I was able to produce the light within and become lost in it for a considerable length of time. I found no difficulty in producing the Shadow Man, so I knew I was ready for the conscious release of the psychic force of man.

The Maharishi gave me the necessary instructions, so I might prepare for the initiation. There were Mantras I should have to use, and a few ritual formalities with which I was already familiar. The practices of Hatha Yoga with which I had been working were designed physically to awaken this power.

This particular initiation has probably less ritual to

it than any other. After the student has made his oblations to his Guru, who is supposed to establish an inner conscious contact between them so he can guide the workings of his pupil's mind, the student then through his imagination mentally tries to awaken Kundalini.

It is taught that in the Kali Yuga man has lost so much of his vital force he has no longer the mental capacity to accomplish this release. A Guru, who is highly developed, must help him. But first it is essential that the student go through the arduous training of Yoga in order to build up sufficient vitality and will power as well as to prepare the body to receive this power when it is released. Under other conditions, there is great danger of insanity or even death on the release of the Power. The various tests given me showed my Guru I was ready.

2

The day arrived. For twenty-four hours I had been on a complete fast. Throughout the day I directed all my meditations towards preparing my mind for the initiation that night. At 10 p.m. I began my Puja (worship), which was for the purpose of fully awakening the heart.

On arriving at the shrine that had been prepared, I took a bath before entering. At the entrance I made my oblation of humility. I drew a triangle and outside it I made a circle. Outside the circle I drew a square. In the centre I placed my vessel and with scented flowers I worshipped the Fire, the Sun, and the Moon in the consecrated water of the vessel. I threw perfume and flowers into the water and recited Mantras while making different Mudras (symbolic mystic gestures) with my hands. These Mudras consist of special formations of the fingers, hands, and wrists.

Picking up my articles of worship, I stepped across the sacred threshold with the left foot, lightly striking my left shoulder on the doorway. First I worshipped before the presiding deity of this Chakra or Shrine.

My Final Initiation

Then I went to the place where I was to worship, and sprinkled it with water taken from the common vessel.

While doing Trataka and repeating what is known as the Weapon-Mantra I sprinkled water to remove all the celestial obstacles, next to remove all the obstacles between heaven and earth and finally to remove all earthly obstacles—this by striking my heel on the floor three times. Filling the place with the incense of burning sandal, saffron, and camphor, I marked off a rectangular space for my seat. After drawing a triangle within it and worshipping, I placed my mat over it and assumed the Padmasana position, facing north. During this my Guru sat motionless.

I did not go through these many ritual formalities as artificially as it seems when described on paper. It was as if some other power was not only directing my actions but controlling my feelings. The various Mantras caused me to lose conscious recognition of my environment and the acts which I was performing. Occasionally my Guru would repeat a Mantra and its rhythm would hold me as spellbound as a great symphony.

After assuming my posture, I went through the rites of purifying my offering, which consisted of the narcotic, Bhang, prepared from the leaves of hemp. As a part of the consecration ceremony I had to recite the Mulamantra over it seven times, and to make various Mudras. When it was consecrated, I then offered it to the residing deity within my head and heart, and finally to the mouth of the Kundalini, all the while uttering Mantras and forming mystic gestures.

After reciting the Mantra composed of words of praise to the Kundalini, I drank of the narcotic and bowed to my Guru by placing my folded hands first on my left ear, then on the right ear and finally on the middle of my forehead; at the same time I sat silently for a few minutes in meditation. Placing the articles of worship on my right side and the wine on my left side, I sprinkled them with water and then encircled myself

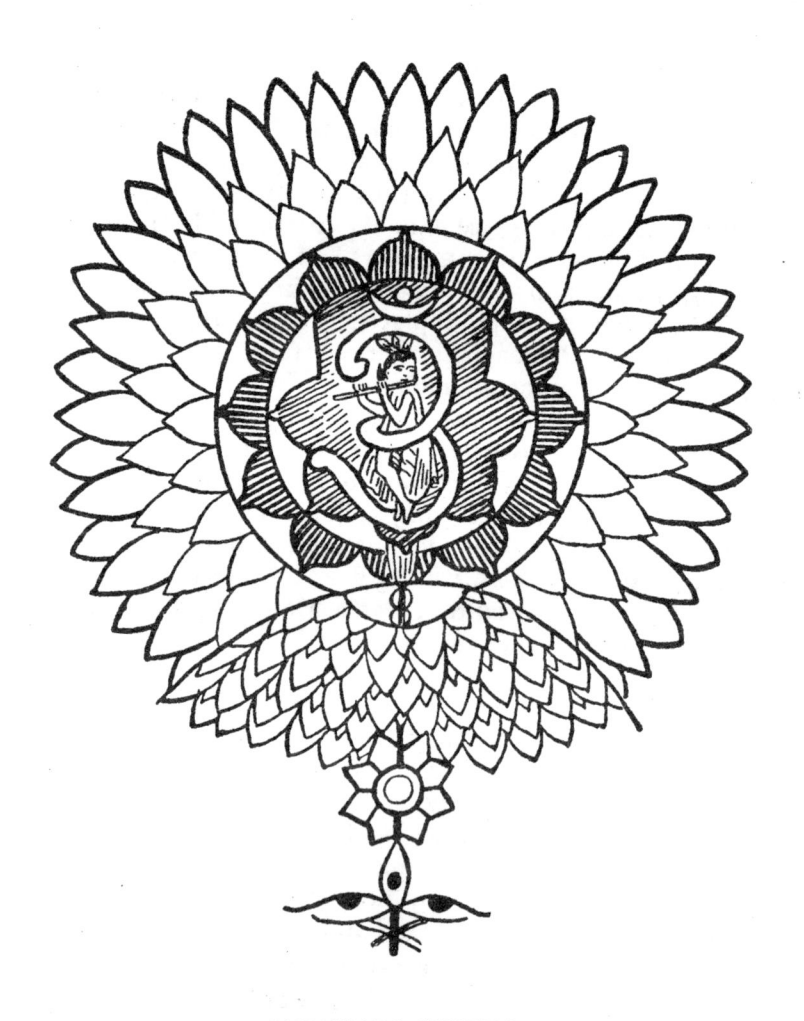

SAHASRARA CHAKRA

My Final Initiation

with water. Then, mentally, I surrounded myself with a wall of Symbolic Fire, after which I purified the palms of my hands by rubbing between them a flower that had been dipped in sandal paste and throwing it over my left shoulder.

As a final protection, I guarded myself from possible evils approaching from the four directions by snapping the thumb and first finger in the palm of the left hand three times. I repeated this in each of the four quarters. Now I was ready to purify the elements of the body which enables the Kundalini to unite with its divine source. Still sitting in the Padmasana posture and placing my folded palms in my lap, I remained silent for a few minutes in order to stable the mind and direct it on the Kundalini. In the process I performed Kumbhaka and followed it with Jalandhara and Aswini Mudra. What happened in that interval must forever remain a mystery—even for me. I shall never know whether I was living in reality or in a state of superconsciousness. I actually had the physical experience of visualizing as well of feeling the awakening of some Divine Power. And from that point onward I could no longer tell whether I was imagining myself to be guiding this force, or whether the experience was actually taking place.

I had been instructed mentally to arouse the Kundalini, which I was to conduct from the Muladhara Chakra by means of Mantras through the other Chakras of the body, the Svadhishthana Manipura, Anahata Vishuddha, and Ajna, finally dissolving this force in the Ahangkara which is the Ego aspect of Consciousness, or the first birth of Self-consciousness.

The faculty of Consciousness was then to be dissolved into the Mahat, which is the formation of the Great Impersonal Intelligence, the first evolute in the growth of the Universe. Then the Mahat was to be dissolved into Prakriti. This is the undifferentiated cosmic substance, the cause of the Universe, often referred to as the "Great Mother," in which all things exist. Finally,

Prakriti itself was to be dissolved into Brahman, which is the First Cause, the unknowable and the unqualified.

Each of these stages was as much a reality to my inner self as any emotional ecstacy that I had ever experienced while sitting on the brink of an Arizona mountain cliff and watching the evening shadows dance on the sun-baked desert, even while the sun was still aglow with its last array of splendour. So often, in those remote days, I had lingered in the emotional awe of the parting day, while I pondered on the nature of things. And now all seemed to have been revealed to me ; I had become one with the Universal Consciousness of Life.

Whether I was under the influence of the narcotic, or in a self-induced trance, or under the hypnotic control of my Guru is still a mystery to me. I do know, however, that at no time was I wholly unconscious. There was an inner awareness, which never once left me. I had the feeling of being under the influence of some mystic light. I was conscious of its unremitting, penetrating, warm rays. This state had come over me rather gradually. Slowly I began to lose track of the path that my imagination was taking. There was a restful dawn of a soft glow. I was held by the awe of it and, as with the sun, there was no cessation of its light. Indeed, its brilliance increased, and its intensity grew more penetrating.

The element of Time had vanished. I had lost consciousness of my external environment. In the midst of all, something snapped, and all was quiet. The light was still there, and I had become absorbed in it. I could no longer find its source. All was light. And I was light. All was peace.

Soon there came flickerings of consciousness and memories of my purpose. The light was fading, my awareness was increasing. I had to return. The memory of my purpose was becoming stronger. After bathing the entire body in this light, I was to seal it within me forever by a series of repetitions of Mantras. After this, with my imagination, I was to carry this light back

My Final Initiation

through all the centres of the body and return the Kundalini to the Muladhara Chakra, where it ever abides in happiness.

The return to my conscious faculties was gradual. I was then to reflect for a short while upon the fact that I had fully realized the identity of the individual and Brahman, or the complete Union of the Individual Consciousness with the Universal Consciousness. There was no longer any doubt in my mind. No sophistry could ever dispel the mood of this conscious experience.

3

A new day had come. In its dawn, the Maharishi, by a twinkle in his eye, silently spoke to me.

It was time to leave. I readily realized that hours had passed when I started to unfold my legs. They had become so numb that I was no longer aware that they belonged to me. I did not want to let the Maharishi know what physical agony I was suffering at the moment. He probably knew what mental experiences had been mine, but I thought I would try to conceal my physical discomfort. So by finessing, with reverent decorum, I slowly began to unfold my legs. Once I had them straightened out, I cautiously rose to a standing position. I did not dare move, as I still had no command of them. It must have been five minutes before it was possible for me to stroll pompously away.

This morning was an exception to my regular practice. The Maharishi, the Swamaji, my Tantrik friend and I were to have breakfast together. It was in the nature of a quiet celebration. During the intervening hour I took my regular stroll over the path which had become so intimate with my inner reflections. On reaching the top of the small knoll, I sat down to reflect.

I felt very much like one who has experienced his first love. I wanted to be alone so I could relive the entire experience.

Something had happened to my inner consciousness, which I was certain would be mine forever. I felt an infinitely greater zest for life. From that moment it coloured all my deeper feelings. My energy seemed inexhaustible. It was no longer going to be a question of being able to find a way to increase my energy. My only future concern would be how to direct it. I now had everything. The question was how to use it.

As I try now to write of this experience. I find it impossible fully to recapture it in words because of the limitation of the name and form which serve as tools. This experience was beyond the mind. It is not so much that it was of such a personal nature that I choose not to speak of it more fully, as that it was so dramatic I am lost for words to express it. To analyse it so that others would fully understand would take volumes, I should have to go into every avenue of human emotion.

If the reader has followed my quest through the maze of discipline and technique, I can, perhaps, best express myself by saying that I found far more than I had hoped for in the beginning. At the beginning my imagination was so undeveloped that it was beyond its power to hold the vaguest idea of the potentialities of human happiness. My early conceptions of happiness were limited. This was one instance when the realization far exceeded the expectation.

The sun had lifted and my friends had gathered. So I hastened back to the dwelling of the Maharishi. It took some time for me emotionally to return to reality, but as the conversation led around to my future plans, my Tantrik friend pointed out that I was no longer dependent on externals to produce the Inner Union. I had perfected this instrument in which I lived and I could produce the static Union at will. I was now free and could find solace in any spot, whether it be Tombstone or Tibet.

4

This did not mean that I was to shun the world. The initiation had given me a realization of the Unity of all things. No longer was there any division between body

My Final Initiation

and spirit. All was one consciousness manifesting itself through an infinity of forms. It was my privilege not only intellectually to see but intuitively to feel the presence of that Universal Consciousness in Matter.

It was pointed out to me that a complete Union with Reality could be accomplished only by a complete Union of the Spirit with Matter. I was not to shun the physical world, for that world was part of the cosmic. It was not I who needed to eat and drink. It was the Divine Shakti who ate and drank through me. Therefore I must not pursue the activities of life egotistically, but always for the Universal Consciousness within me.

For me to neglect or deny the needs of the body would be to neglect or deny that consciousness. It was for me to realize the cosmic consciousness in even the lowest physical needs. The body with all its needs is a manifestation of the Divine, and the way for me to realize it fully was by perfecting my personal potentialities, yet not becoming lost in the Ego which is merely the conscious instrument for direction. This I was to do by living, which meant returning to ordinary life and yet making that life the Real Life at its fullest. This time intelligence must rule. Since all life is illusory, it is only through the full understanding of suffering that man can gain the true wisdom which liberates. The bliss of liberation can be gained here when the identity of all things is realized. This may be achieved by making every human function an act of sacrifice. It is wrong to believe that happiness can be gained only in the hereafter.

All is one. The physical, mental, and spiritual can never be separated. They are merely different aspects of the One. The development of one aspect is the development of the others. The way fully to awaken consciousness is to live.

He who is so Holy that he spurns the body is lost in his own Ego. Realization will come only by discerning the Spirit in every activity. The way of Man is to Live. Intelligent living is the Instrument of God. All actions will give enjoyment when done with the right feeling and right frame of mind. If this is repeated and prolonged enough, it will in the end produce the divine experience of Liberation.

I had learned to Live.

Having a desire to learn more of the philosophy which lies behind the practice of Yoga, I inquired again where it would be possible for me to secure the manuscripts of the Sixty-four Tantras. Tibet, was the answer. This was like saying that they could be found in "Heaven," for Tibet is a Forbidden Land, and even the few travallers who had crossed its windswept plateaus had been permitted to learn only of the material aspects of the culture. No one had ever been allowed to dip into the consciousness of these people and learn of their jealously guarded teachings.

The Maharishi smiled when I said I would go.

This was enough for me. I saw I had his confidence. Immediately plans were made for me to leave for the border of Tibet, where I was to continue my Yoga discipline, and begin to learn the Tibetan language, letting the guiding hand of Fate take care of the rest. This experience I have related in my book: *Land of a Thousand Buddhas*.

5

THE parting words of the Maharishi were:

"Return to your world and give an intellectual grasp of your realization to the candidates for humanity."

INDEX

Abdominal control, 31
Abstraction, 104
Acquired mark, 228
Adharkunda, 137
Adhikara, 25
Agni, 139, 152, 208, 234, 238
Ahangkara, 247
Ajna Chakra, 83, 247
Akasha, 139, 140
Amabashya, 137
Anahata, 139, 227, 242
Anahata Vishudda, 242, 247
Apana, 134, 140, 199, 206, 208, 209, 239
Apas, 139, 157
Artha, 22
Asanas, 27 et seq., 58, 60, 148, 166, 180 et seq.
Asanas, Spiritual and Physical, 181
Asanas, thirty-two, 180
Aswini Mudra, 199 et seq., 206, 207 213, 236, 239-241
Atma, 96

Baddha-Padmasana, 239
Basti, 42, 43, 123, 198, 200 et seq., 232
Beck, Adams, 17
Beetle-droning Kumbhaka, 240
Behanan, Dr. Kovoor T., 120
Benares, 116, 120
Bhadrasana, 180
Bhakti Yoga, 75
Bhastrika Kumbhaka, 158, 160-163, 195, 231, 239
Bhedas, 157
Bhramari Kumbhaka, 240
Bhujangasana, 180
Bhujangini, 206
Bija Mantra, 236
Bindu, 209, 234
Bombay, 120 et seq.
Brahma Granthi, 163
Brahma Nadi, 163, 234
Brahman, 248
Brahman, union with, 249
Brahmarandra, 208, 236
Breath Alternation, 140-141

Breath Control (vide Pranayama)
Breath Rhythmic, 92

Calcutta, 48 et seq., 170 et seq.
Cardiac plexus, 100
Chakra, 87, 206, 236-238, 244, 247
Chastity, 65, 147
Chaturvarga, 22
Chhaya Pursha Sadhana, 222 et seq.
Chitta, 100, 107 et seq., 217, 241
Chitta and Prana, 108
Chittra, 83
Concentration, 104, 107 et seq., 219 228
Consciousness, 99 et seq.
Contemplation, 104
Contemplation, luminous, 224
Crow Bill Mudra, 161

Delhi, 116, 120
Devadatta, 134
Dhanamiaya, 134
Dhanurasana, 180
Dharana, 58 et seq., 242
Dharma, 21, 22, 59
Dhatus, 152
Dhyana, 58, 61, 105, 215, 242
Dhyana Yoga, 75
Diet, 59, 73, 126, 197, 217, 230, 238 239, 241
Divine Body of Truth, 226
Divya, 22
Door of Brahma, 82
Doshas, three, 148
Dvapara Yuga, 21
Dying at will, 150

Ecstacy of living, 195
Enema and Basti, 43, 202

Fire Meditation, 224
First Breath, 134
Five Elements, 242
Frontal Gaze, 225

Gallhuber, J., quoted 101
Garudasana, 180
Gheranda Samhita, 180, 204

Index

Gomukhasana, 180
Goraksasana, 180
Grand Potential, 233
Great Mother, 248
Gunas, three, 104
Gunas and Samadhi, 104
Guptasana, 180
Guru and Chela, 169

Halasana, 183
Hatha Yoga, 74, 77, 79, 102, 227, 229, 232, 239, 243
Head stand, 193 et seq., 231
Heavenly passage (vide Reissner)
Higher self, 107, 122
Holy Man of Hyderabad, 122

Ida, 137, 151, 187, 188, 219, 238
Initiation, 87 et seq., 229, 243 et seq.
Intellect v. intelligence, 97

Jalandhara, 105, 128, 148, 158, 165, 204, 206, 207, 209, 236, 238, 240
Japa, 166
Jiva, 59, 134
Jnana Yoga, 75

Kaki Mudra, 161, 206
Kali Yuga, 20, 55, 150, 244
Kama, 23
Kapalabahati, 41, 43, 123, 154, 155, 161
Kapha, 20, 41, 82, 148, 154, 191
Karma builds Chitta, 108
Karma Yoga, 75
Kevala Kumbhaka, 241
Khecari, 41, 191, 196, 202, 204, 207, 231, 238, 241
Krita, 21
Krkara, 134
Kukkutsana, 180
Kulanarva Tantra, 65
Kumbhaka, 126–128, 145, 149, 150, 152, 158, 159, 160, 161, 165, 166, 206, 207, 209, 210, 212, 236, 238, 240
Kumbhaka and Samadhi, 130
Kumbhaka, Greater, 129
Kundalini, 83, 129, 137, 155, 157, 158, 160, 163, 187, 200, 204, 206, 208, 210, 211, 224, 230 et seq.
Kundalini, Awakening, 238 et seq., 244
Kundalini Yoga, 75
Kurmasana, 180

Laya Yoga, 74, 78, 226 *et seq.*

Levitation by Pranayama, 149, 152, 167
Liberation (vide Moksha)
Life Coil, 135
Linga Sharira, 140
Living on air, 129
Lotus Pose (vide Padmasana)

Madras, 122
Mahabandha, 204, 208, 209
Mahamudra, 204, 206, 208
Mahat, 247
Mahavadasa Basti, 200
Mahavedha, 204, 209
Makarasana, 180
Manduka Mudra, 159, 204, 208, 211
Mandukasana, 180
Manipura Chakra, 139, 163, 242
Mantras, 59, 74, 77, 152, 236 et seq.
Manu, laws of, 21
Matangi, 206
Matsyasana, 180
Matsyendrasana, 180
Maya, 145
Mayurasana, 180, 183, 201
Meditation, 105, 106, 217 et seq.
Mental Development, stages of, 104
Mental States, five, 97
Mind and Breathing, 91 et seq
Mind Control, obstacles to, 103
Mind v. Intellect, 97
Mind, Yogic view of, 90 et seq.
Moksha, 23, 227
Moon Breath (vide Ida)
Mritasana, 149, 180
Mudras, 199 et seq, 204 et seq, 244
Muktasana, 180
Mulabandha, 105, 129, 204, 208, 209, 236
Muladhara, 137, 139, 209, 234, 239, 242, 247
Mulamantra, 245
Murchchha Kumbhaka, 241
Mysore, 166 et seq.
Mysterious Kundalini, The, 121

Nabo Mudra, 204, 207
Nada, 234
Nadis, 82, 83, 139, 148, 154, 156, 158, 166, 204, 207, 208, 211, 222, 227, 234, 238
Naga, 134
Nasagra Drishti, 225
Nasal Gaze, 225
Nauli, 30, 31, 34, 41, 123, 192, 198, 200 et seq., 213, 239, 240
Nerve Centres, five, 139
Nerve Control (vide Pratyahara)

Nerve Culture, 80
Neti, 41, 45, 123, 191
Nirvana, 24, 108
Niyama, 58, 59

Ojuh, 212, 228

Padmasana, 27, 34, 60, 124, 157, 161, 165, 181-184, 186, 194, 197, 210, 238, 245
Pancadharana, 204
Patanjali, 61
Paschini, 206
Paschimottanasana, 180, 183
Pashu, 22
Peacock Pose (vide Mayurasana)
Perfect Pose, 184
Pingala, 137, 142, 152, 187, 188, 219, 238
Pitta, 148, 163, 165
Postures (vide Asanas)
Prakriti, 233, 247
Prana, 82, 90, 91, 94, 96, 98, 134-136, 138-140, 150, 152, 208, 209, 211, 224, 227, 236-238
Prana Gopala Tapani Upanishad, 140
Prana Wayu, 105, 208, 209, 212
Pranayama, 58, 60, 77, 80, 82, 94, 123, 125, 129, 133, 145, 147, 148, 149, 150, 152, 156, 159, 160, 168, 187, 191, 194, 197, 203, 204, 208, 211, 227, 229, 231, 242
PranayamaTechnique, 123 et seq., 131
Pratyahara, 58, 60, 80, 153
Prithivi, 139, 157
Prosperous Pose, 187
Puraka, 145, 154, 155, 166
Puranas, 21
Purification, physical, 41 et seq.

Rajaguna, 104, 233
Raja Yoga, 58, 78
Rasa, 152, 168
Rasananda-Yoga Samadhi, 240
Rechaka, 145, 154, 155, 166
Reissner Passage, 83
Rele, Vasant G., 121
Rudra Granthi, 163

Sadhaka, 41, 146, 232
Sadhaka Titta, 151
Sadhana, 41
Sages, peaceful aura of, 178
Sahita Kumbhaka, 165
Samadhi, 58, 61, 104, 105, 150, 152, 236, 241, 242
Samadhi Yoga, 75

Samana, 134, 140, 206, 208
Samana Wayu, 209
Samkatasana, 180
Samyama, 242
Sarvangasana, 148, 181
Sattwa Guna, 104, 226, 233
Satya Yuga, 21
Science of Breath, 133 et seq.
Science of Tattvas, 136
Scientific Evaluation of Yoga, 120
Seed Mantras, 236
Semen, Mind and Prana, 211
Serpent Power, 121
Serpent Power (vide also Kundalini), 210
Sex Control, 212
Shadow Man, 222, 229
Shakti, 134, 152, 227
Shaktichalana, 204, 236, 239, 241
Shakti Nadi, 163
Shakti Yoga, 75
Shalabhasana, 180
Shambhavi Mudra, 204, 211, 224
Shatkarmas, 41 et seq.
Shri Paramahatma Sachitananda Yogiswarar, 122 et seq.
Siddhasana, 60, 124, 157, 161, 180-182, 186, 188, 208, 212, 225, 226, 238-241
Siddhis, 224, 237
Simhasana, 180
Sirshasana, 32 et seq., 183
Sitali, 157-160, 165
Sitkari, 159, 165
Sleep and Tamas, 151
Smritis, 21
Srimat Kuvalayananda, 120
Stages of Training, Six, 67
Story of Philosophy, 17
Sukhasana, 181
Sukshma Dhyana, 224
Sun Breath (vide Pingala)
Sun and Moon Breaths, 137
Supine Pelvic Posture, 189
Supreme Bliss, 104, 106
Supta Vajrasana, 189
Surya, 157
Suryabheda Kumbhaka, 157, 158, 165
Sushumna, 82, 168, 187, 206, 207, 234, 236, 238, 239
Svadisthana Chakra, 138, 139, 239, 242
Svadisthana Manipura, 247
Swara Shastra, 136
Swarodaya, 134, 138
Swastikasana, 60, 180, 181, 186-188
Sympathetic System, 83

Index

Tadagi, 204
Tamaguna, 104, 233
Tantras, 21, 23, 83, 84, 252
Tantrik Teachers, Tibetan, 84
Tattwas, 136, 138, 140, 157, 210, 211, 227
Tattwas, Rise of, 187, 204
Tattwic Changes, 138
Thousand-Petalled Lotus, 105, 236
Thunderbolt Posture, 188
Trataka, 41, 43, 123, 221, 229, 245
Treta Yuga, 21
Trivarga, 24

Udana, 134, 135, 140
Uddiyana, 28 *et seq.*, 34, 105, 192, 198-200, 204, 206, 213, 224, 236, 239, 240
Uddiyana Bandha, 206, 239, 240
Ujjayi, 157, 158, 165
Unmani, 125, 225
Unmani Mudra, 224
Upanishads, 21, 140
Ushtrasana, 180
Utkasana, 180
Uttama Pranayama, 167
Uttana Kurmakasana, 180
Uttana Mandukasana, 180

Vagus Nerve, 150
Vajrasana, 60, 161, 180, 181, 188, 189
Vajroli, 204, 211-213, 232
Vaschaspti, quoted, 149
Vedanta Sara, 182

Vedas, 21
Viparitakarani, 204
Vira, 22
Virasana, 180
Visions, 222
Vishnu Granthi, 163
Vishudda, 139, 242
Vital Air (*vide* also Prana), 135, 136, 140
Vow of Secrecy, 35, 87
Vrikshasana, 180
Vrishasana, 180
Vyana, 134, 140

Wadda Padmasana, 186
Water Centre, 239
Wayu, 134, 139, 148, 151, 163, 165, 168, 207, 213, 234, 238
Wayu Siddhi, 188, 209
Weapon Mantra, 245
Wisdom *v.* Learning, 62
Woodroffe, Sir John, 121
Writtis, 107, 108

Yama, 58, 59
Yantra Yoga, 75
Yantram, 39
Yoga, seventeen meanings of, 52-53; six obstacles to, 57, 61; three aims of, 54; eight limbs of, 58; seven ethical requirements, 58; mystical aspects of, 215 *et seq.*
Yoga Mudra, 210
Yogasana, 180
Yoni Mudra, 204, 209, 239